D0773195

Understanding Periodontal Diseases
Assessment and Diagnostic Procedures in Practice

Understanding Periodontal Diseases Assessment and Diagnostic Procedures in Practice

By
Iain L C Chapple and Angela D Gilbert

Editor-in-Chief: Nairn H F Wilson
Editor Periodontology: Iain L C Chapple

Quintessence Publishing Co. Ltd.

London, Berlin, Chicago, Copenhagen, Paris, Milan, Barcelona,
Istanbul, São Paulo, Tokyo, New Dehli, Moscow, Prague, Warsaw

British Library Cataloguing in Publication Data

Chapple, Iain L. (Iain Leslie)
Understanding periodontal diseases: assessment and diagnostic procedures in
practice. - (The quintessentials of dental practice)
1. Periodontal disease - Diagnosis 2. Periodontal disease - Treatment
I. Title II. Gilbert, Angela D. III. Wilson, Nairn H. F. 617.6'32

1-85097-053-X

ISBN 1-85097-053-X

This text is dedicated to my daughter,
Jessica Louise Chapple, born 7 September 2001.

Iain L C Chapple

Foreword

Knowledge and understanding of the periodontal tissues and diseases are fundamental to the provision of effective oral healthcare. This first volume in the Quintessentials for General Dental Practitioners Series presents this knowledge and understanding in a succinct, authoritative, easy-to-read engaging style.

Each chapter includes aims, anticipated outcomes, high-quality illustrations to complement the text and carefully selected suggestions for further reading - features which will characterise the attractive range of books to follow in the Quintessentials Series. As a rich mine of information and guidance essential to good-quality periodontology in everyday clinical practice, *Understanding Periodontal Diseases* has a good deal to offer both established practitioners of all ages and student members of the dental team.

With a growing awareness of the benefits of oral health, patients living longer and retaining an increasing number of teeth throughout life, periodontology as presented in *Understanding Periodontal Diseases* is an essential element of successful clinical practice. For all those striving to improve the provision of oral healthcare for their patients, this book, in common with the volumes to follow in the Quintessentials Series, provides a most valuable asset - the means for all practitioners to apply the latest knowledge and understanding for the benefit of patients and the further development of the art and science of dentistry. I commend *Understanding Periodontal Diseases* to you as an outstanding first volume in the Quintessentials for Dental Practitioners Series.

Nairn H F Wilson
Editor-in-Chief

Preface

This text is the first of five books which aim to provide the general dental practitioner with an illustrated practical and contemporary guide to the management of patients with gingival and periodontal diseases. The first book in the series is entitled *Understanding Periodontal Diseases: Assessment and Diagnostic Procedures in Practice* and takes the reader on a logical journey through the assessment and diagnostic processes to enable practitioners to avoid diagnostic pitfalls and to identify *risk patients* for periodontitis. It provides summary background revision of anatomical issues and those relating to the disease process, clinical signs of health and disease and current concepts of disease classification. The reader is then led through a clinical diagnostic algorithm, including radiological and other special investigations and is provided with a look into the future for periodontal diagnosis.

Having Read This Book

It is hoped that having read this book the reader will be able to:
- Understand current concepts of the periodontal disease process, its classification and clinical course.
- Understand the concept of risk assessment and what risk factors are, and be able to assign a level of risk for their patients losing teeth due to periodontitis.
- Identify healthy and diseased periodontal tissues, in their broadest sense, and understand how such features fit into current classification systems.
- Diagnose the most common gingival and periodontal diseases/lesions.
- Follow a simple periodontal diagnostic algorithm, including radiological and other special investigations, thereby ensuring that disease does not go undetected.
- Decide on the most appropriate radiographs to take and to prepare and document a concise report of the key findings from such investigations.
- Understand which special tests are required for certain conditions and what the results mean.
- Broadly categorise lesions affecting the periodontal tissues and form differential diagnoses for such conditions.
- Picture where periodontal diagnosis may be heading over the next ten years and therefore prepare their practice for potential change.

Iain L C Chapple
Angela D Gilbert

Acknowledgements

The authors would like to acknowledge with sincere thanks the following people. Dr John Strange and Dr Barbara Shearer for proof-reading the entire manuscript; Dr John Matthews for proof-reading Chapters 2 and 3; Mr Michael Sharland and Miss Marina Tipton for their photographic expertise; Dr Rachel Sammons for Figs 2-2, 2-3, 2-4, 2-5, 3-7; Mr H Donald Glenwright for the use of Fig 4-9; Dr John Rippin for the use of Figs 1-1, 1-4, 1-5; Dr Serge Dibart for the use of Figs 1-7 and 5-8; Dr Elizabeth Connor and her staff for radiological expertise and material; Mr Paul Hughes for his help with illustrations and Mosby Year Book Europe Limited for allowing us to reprint Figs 6-2 and 6-4.

Professor Chapple would like to acknowledge the help and support of his wife, Liz, throughout this venture. Dr Gilbert would like to thank Nigel, and her sisters Isobell and Joan for their unstinting support.

Contents

Chapter 1
A Whistle-Stop Tour of the Periodontium

Aim

This chapter aims to provide the practitioner with a contemporary review of the important anatomical and micro-anatomical features of the periodontium.

Outcome

At the end of this chapter the practitioner should be able to identify key clinical features that need to be assessed during the examination of patients' periodontal tissues, since these features help inform diagnostic and treatment-planning processes.

Terminology and Orientation

The periodontal tissues form the supporting apparatus of the teeth. Their role is to protect the teeth from masticatory forces and infection, thereby facilitating normal oral function and preventing premature tooth loss. As modern medicine and standards of health have prolonged human life expectancy the periodontal tissues have to perform these functions over considerably more years than they were designed for, and therefore recession, sensitivity and tooth mobility are daily management problems for the dental practitioner and patient. Additionally, the nature and extent of systemic problems that are created by a compromised periodontal attachment (e.g. the established link between periodontal disease and cardio-/cerebro-vascular disease) and the chronic microbial stimulus associated with retaining teeth for longer, is only just being realised. The healthy periodontal tissues are identified in Fig 1-1 and comprise:

- investing gingival complex (gingivae)
- alveolar bone
- periodontal ligament
- root cementum.

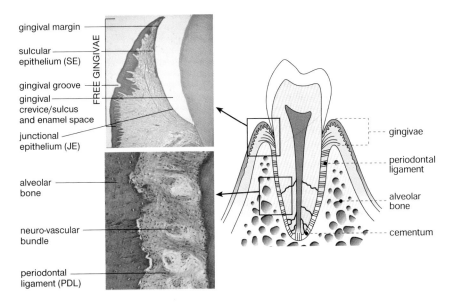

Fig 1-1 Schematic longitudinal section of a premolar and associated periodontal tissues. Applied anatomy is demonstrated alongside histology (photomicrographs) of key areas.

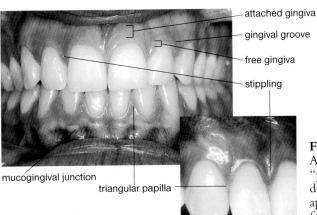

Fig 1-2
An anterior view of "pristine gingivae" demonstrating applied anatomical features from Fig 1-1.

The Gingivae

The gingivae comprise:
- a gingival margin – the visible edge of the gingiva
- a gingival sulcus – (or crevice) which in health is between 0.5 and 3mm in depth

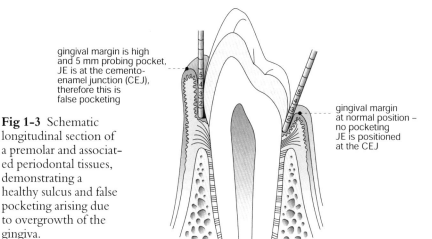

gingival margin is high and 5 mm probing pocket, JE is at the cemento-enamel junction (CEJ), therefore this is false pocketing

gingival margin at normal position – no pocketing JE is positioned at the CEJ

Fig 1-3 Schematic longitudinal section of a premolar and associated periodontal tissues, demonstrating a healthy sulcus and false pocketing arising due to overgrowth of the gingiva.

- the free gingiva – a mobile cuff of gingiva lying above the alveolar crest
- the attached gingiva – a band of 1–9mm in length, which is bound down to the underlying alveolus and cementum, by collagen fibres of the dentogingival complex.

The line at which the *free gingiva* becomes *attached gingiva* is usually visible, under conditions of *pristine* gingival health, as the *gingival groove* (Figs 1-1 and 1-2). However, since the majority of healthy mouths have detectable levels of marginal and interproximal plaque present, they also have a degree of inflammation present histologically, hence *clinical health* and *pristine health* are now recognised as different conditions. In clinical gingival health, it is accepted that there may be very mild inflammation present and the gingival groove is not therefore always discernible.

The gingival tissues are orthokeratinised and therefore, in health, appear paler or pinker than the lining oral mucosa, which is non-keratinised. The gingiva joins the oral mucosa at the *mucogingival junction* (MGJ), which is not visible in the palate, since palatal mucosa is entirely keratinised. It used to be thought that when the gingival margin was formed by oral mucosa (e.g. due to recession) rather than keratinised gingiva, the marginal tissues were less robust and resistant to the trauma of toothbrushing. However, studies have shown that a gingival margin formed by non-keratinised oral mucosa is as capable of retaining stability as a margin formed by keratinised gingiva, provided plaque control is good.

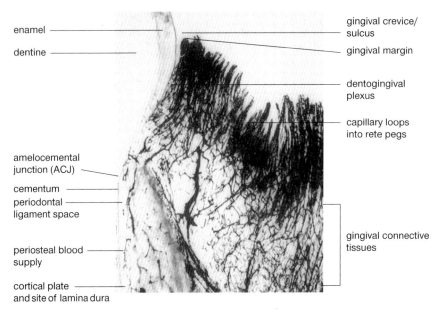

enamel

dentine

amelocemental
junction (ACJ)

cementum

periodontal
ligament space

periosteal blood
supply

cortical plate
and site of lamina dura

gingival crevice/
sulcus

gingival margin

dentogingival
plexus

capillary loops
into rete pegs

gingival connective
tissues

Fig 1-4 A black–and–white photomicrograph from the periodontium of a dog following injection of dye to demonstrate the rich gingival vasculature. Large vessels (arterioles) branch off a vast network of capillaries which form loops beneath the connective tissue rete ridges of the oral epithelium. The capillary network beneath the JE and SE is called the dentogingival plexus and serum from this plexus either returns to the post-capillary venules, or it enters the gingival crevice as GCF.

The free gingival tissues are separated from the crown of the tooth in health by the *gingival sulcus* or crevice, which on clinical probing varies from 0.5 to 3mm, for recommended probing pressures (20–25g or 0.2–0.25N) (Fig 1-3). If a healthy crevice is probed too firmly, the probe penetrates the base and enters the connective tissues. The crevice is washed out in health by *gingival crevicular fluid* (GCF) which flows out at a rate of 0.2μl per hour contributing 1ml per day to saliva. GCF is a serum *transudate* in health and is formed by serum moving passively from the arteriolar capillaries of the gingiva (Fig 1-4), through the gingival connective tissues and into the gingival crevice (Fig 1-5). In health, GCF contains everything serum contains, except for red blood cells, and, in addition, viable neutrophils (polymorphonuclear leucocytes; PMNLs) can be collected from it. During inflammation, the transudate becomes more like an inflammatory *exudate* and local components of that inflammatory process enter the GCF, which increases in flow rate and volume.

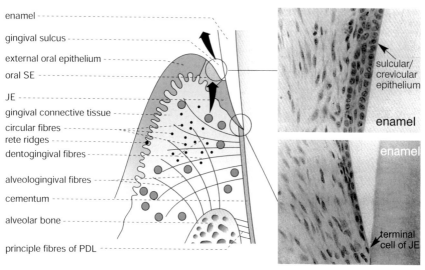

Fig 1-5 A schematic view of the gingivae demonstrating the gingival collagen fibre complexes. The SE and JE are also represented alongside in two photomicrographs demonstrating normal histology. Note how widely spaced the cells are and how they thin out forming a single "terminal cell" of the apex of the JE.

The gingival crevice is lined by highly specialised epithelia called sulcular epithelium (SE) and junctional epithelium (JE) (Fig 1-5). These normally adhere tightly to the crown, such that in *pristine* health no sulcus exists unless a probe is placed down from the gingival margin. The JE is unique as it forms an epithelial attachment (via hemi-desmosomes) to an internalised part of the skeleton (tooth with its investing alveolar bone). As enamel is derived from ectoderm embryologically (inner enamel epithelium) such a union is not unusual. However, once attachment loss has occurred (either recession or true pocket formation), the JE migrates onto cementum which is derived from mesenchyme. This results in a situation rather like a compound fracture of bone, where bone emerges from epithelium exposing the internal structures of the body to a hostile external environment. For this reason, the JE is permeable to GCF carrying the host's defence cells (mainly PMNLs) and various other components of the inflammatory/immune response, such as *complement* and *antibody*. The JE cells are widely spaced to fa-

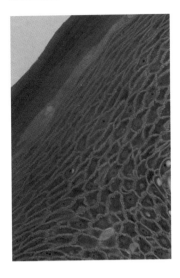

Fig 1-6 Photomicrograph of gingival epithelium from the facial surface demonstrating columnar basal cells (just in view) and pentagonal cells of the stratum spinosum, with flattened surface cells which have accumulated keratin. Note the absence of nuclei at the very surface, which is pure keratin and forms the permeability barrier to prevent microbial invasion. (From Riviere, *Lab Manual of Normal Oral Histology*. Quintessence: Chicago, 2000)

cilitate this (Fig 1-5), but the downside of this arrangement is that bacterial products can also pass back into the gingival tissues and stimulate an inflammatory reaction. In health, this reaction is controlled and visible inflammation does not occur. However, as plaque accumulates subgingivally, the inflammation progresses within the gingival connective tissue underlying the JE and the latter eventually develops microscopic ulcers. When probed, blood can pass from the gingival connective tissues via the micro-ulcerations and can enter the crevice, creating the important clinical sign of *bleeding on probing* (BOP).

The Gingival Epithelium

The gingival epithelium comprises:
- oral epithelium
- oral sulcular/crevicular epithelium
- junctional epithelium.

The oral epithelium (Fig 1-6) is a stratified squamous epithelium with several layers, starting with the columnar basal cells. These germinal cells divide to produce cells that move up to the central zone (pentagonal/hexagonal cells within the *stratum spinosum* and *stratum granulosum*), which ultimately flatten at the surface and lose their nuclei. The surface cells accumulate an impermeable protein called keratin and upon death they lie along the gingival surface forming a non-nucleated and impermeable keratinised layer (orthokeratinisation). There are over 20 different types of keratin and the keratin profile of epithelial cells characterises where they come from (e.g. gingival epithelium expresses cytokeratin – K1, 2, 5, 6, 10, 12, 16). The basal layer of cells follows a "rollercoaster" course as they travel over connective tissue ridges called *"rete ridges"* designed to increase the surface area of epithelial-connective tissue contact. The oral gingival epithelium forms a key part of the innate immune response by forming an impermeable physical barrier to bacteria and their products, which is bathed by saliva containing a variety of enzymes (e.g. lysozyme) and imunoglobulins (antibody). As the oral epithelium drops down inside the gingival margin, it becomes SE.

The SE is midway between the oral epithelium and the JE. There are no rete ridges for the basal cells to conform to (Fig 1-5). The basal layer divides rapidly, increasing turnover of the surface layer to help shed bacteria that attach to epithelial cells within the gingival sulcus. As a result these cells have less time to accumulate keratin and surface cells are para-keratinised (they still have nuclei), eventually losing their keratin surface as they touch the tooth. At this point they become highly specialised JE and express K19 and K13 in addition to the more ubiquitous keratins. Both the sulcular epithelial cells and junctional epithelial cells are "active epithelial cells", capable of pinocytosis of bacteria (Fig 1-7) and production of important cell signalling molecules called cytokines (e.g. interleukin 1 – IL-1), which are chemical messengers that set up early inflammatory changes in the underlying gingival connective tissues.

The JE is a highly specialised epithelial tissue whose cells are non-keratinised and divide faster than any other normal epithelium (2-6-day turnover, compared to a month for oral epithelium). The JE is the key to determining when *gingivitis* becomes *periodontitis*. It is positioned onto enamel in health and, in longitudinal section, tapers from 20 to 30 cells thick to the apical cell of the JE (Fig 1-5), which is a single cell positioned at the CEJ. As the underlying periodontal attachment (ligament and cementum) becomes damaged during early periodontitis, the JE migrates down the root surface in an effort to *wall off* the vital internalised tissues from the potentially hostile bacteria within the crevice and their products. The *apical migration of the JE* is the first clinical indicator of *periodontal attachment loss*, and results in the formation of a *true pocket*. A *false pocket* arises when the gingival margin expands coronally (e.g. with drug-induced gingival overgrowth – Fig 1-3), the crevice deepens beyond 3mm, but the apical cell of the JE remains at the CEJ and

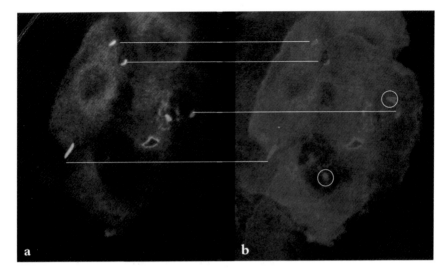

Fig 1-7 (a) A single sulcular epithelial cell curetted from a patient who harboured the pathogen *B.forsythus*. Green fluorescein-labelled secondary antibody raised against *B.forsythus*. Under a microscope with a green filter, the green fluorescein dye labels *B.forsythus* located outside the cell.

(b) Red rhodamine-labelled secondary antibody raised against *B.forsythus* after holes were punched into epithelial cell membrane to allow antibody inside. The red dye stains *B.forsythus* located both inside and outside the cell. Thus, bacteria located outside the cell take up a double label and stain both red and green. Those bacteria located inside the cell stain with the red label only. Note the bacteria inside the epithelial cell appear inside vacuoles after pinocytosis.

there has been no *attachment loss*. A simple formula is used to define the *clinical attachment level* (CAL):

CAL = probing pocket depth + recession

where recession is the distance measured from the CEJ to the gingival margin. If the gingival margin is apical to the CEJ then this is recession; if it is coronal to the CEJ then this is "overgrowth" and false pocketing (Fig 1-3). Clearly, this assumes that the gingival margin is at the CEJ in health, when in fact it lies coronal to the CEJ and is broadly attached by hemidesmosomes up to 2–3mm above the CEJ (Fig 1-1). True recession should be measured from the CEJ to the point of epithelial attachment to the root surface

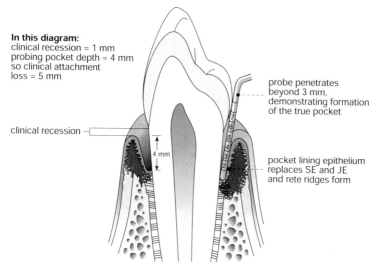

In this diagram:
clinical recession = 1 mm
probing pocket depth = 4 mm
so clinical attachment
loss = 5 mm

clinical recession

4 mm

probe penetrates
beyond 3 mm,
demonstrating formation
of the true pocket

pocket lining epithelium
replaces SE and JE
and rete ridges form

Fig 1-8 Schematic longitudinal section of a premolar and associated periodontal tissues, demonstrating early true pocket formation, detected by probing.

(Fig 1-8), but this is not visible clinically and hence the term "*clinical attachment level*" rather than "*histological attachment level*" is used to overcome this. *Clinical* recession is a visual gap between the gingival margin and CEJ and *clinical* pocketing is measured by probing (hence the term probing pocket depth (PPD), rather than *true* pocket depth). It can also be seen that what represents the "normal" position of the gingival margin and what represents "overgrowth" are open to clinical interpretation.

The interdental papilla covers the interdental bone crest and is a fragile structure due to the anatomy of its blood supply, where buccal and lingual micro-vessels meet in a narrow isthmus. In health the papilla shape is determined by the tooth contacts, and it is normally triangular (pyramidal in 3-dimensions) due to tight tooth contacts (Fig 1-2). However, if the teeth are spaced apart, the triangularity is lost (Fig 1-9), but the tissue may still be healthy. Where the facial and lingual papillae meet within the interdental zone, is a "*col*", situated beneath the contact point of the tooth. This area is the most vulnerable to disease initiation and progression, as the epithelium is non-keratinised and the col-area difficult to access for oral hygiene (very few people routinely clean interproximally). As a result of this, gingival inflammation tends to initiate in this area and interdental bone loss follows.

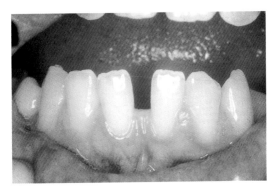

Fig 1-9 Clinical photograph of healthy gingivae, demonstrating the effect of the tooth contact area in dictating interdental papilla shape. The schematic diagrams show the narrow contact point and narrow col between incisors and the broader contact and deeper, more vulnerable col area between molar teeth.

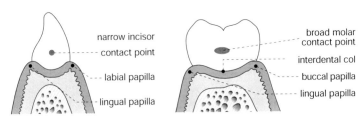

The Gingival Connective Tissues

The gingival connective tissues essentially comprise ground substance, blood and lymph vessels and neural tissue, transsected by a series of collagenous fibre bundles called the *gingival fibres*. The latter comprise:
- dentogingival fibres (Fig 1-5)
- alveolar-gingival fibres (or alveolar crest fibres) – (Fig 1-5)
- circumferential fibres (circular or circum-gingival fibres) – (Fig 1-5)
- transeptal fibres (or interdental fibres) – (Fig 1-10).

The main cells present are fibroblasts which produce collagen and the collagenases to replace collagen, and, even in health, some inflammatory cells (PMNLs, monocytes, T- and B-lymphocytes). The purpose of the gingival fibres is to maintain a tight gingival cuff and close adaptation of gingiva to tooth, restricting subgingival microbial colonisation. When the gingivae become inflamed, they fill with inflammatory exudate (oedema), blood vessels dilate, and the fibres become stretched resulting in the gingivae loosening, and becoming rounded and swollen (see Chapter 5).

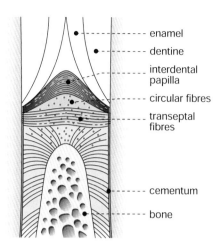

enamel

dentine

interdental
papilla

circular fibres

transeptal
fibres

cementum

bone

Fig 1-10 Schematic facial view of the interdental area showing the transeptal fibres and cross-section of the circular fibres.

The Periodontal Attachment Apparatus

The periodontal attachment apparatus describes:
- root cementum – which normally finishes at the CEJ but can extend onto enamel
- periodontal ligament (PDL) – which is 0.2mm wide in health
- alveolar bone – that part of the mandible or maxilla that forms the tooth socket.

Root cementum
The cementum is a bone-like tissue (approximately 50% mineral, but containing no blood, lymph or neural structures) that covers the root and protects the root dentine from collagenases released by periodontal fibroblasts. But importantly it anchors the ends of the PDL fibres to the root. It is thinner at the coronal end (about 0.05–0.1mm by CEJ) and becomes thicker towards the tooth apex (around 0.2–1mm). There are two types of cementum:

- acellular cementum – forms next to the root dentine during tooth development and forms around the inserting fibres of the PDL which are called *Sharpey's fibres* at this point (Fig 1-11).
- cellular cementum – contains cementocytes in lacunae and forms during function on the surface of acellular cementum

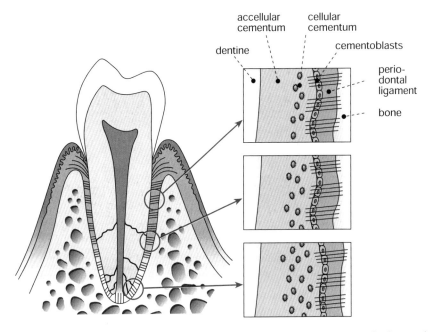

Fig 1-11 Schematic view of basic cementum structure. Note towards the tooth apex the cementum layer becomes thicker and more cellular.

Theoretically, the cementum should finish at the CEJ (Fig 1-12), but it can lie just short (Fig 1-13) or have deficiencies within (cemental tears) or may even overlie the enamel (Fig 1-14). It is the surface of cementum that bacterial endotoxin (or lipopolysaccharide – LPS) loosely attaches to in the diseased pocket. Root surface debridement (RSD) aims to remove the infected cementum layer (top 10–15%) or to wash out endotoxin from its surface using ultrasonic or sonic scalers.

PDL
The PDL is a more dynamic structure than cementum and is approximately 0.2–0.4mm wide, reaching from a point 1.5mm apical to the CEJ and investing the entire root surface. The PDL comprises the following:

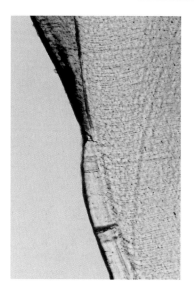

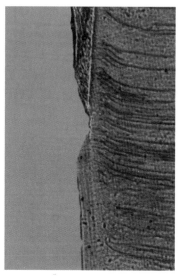

Fig 1-12 Photomicrograph of "normal" cementum position relative to the CEJ (30% of cases). (From Riviere, *Lab Manual of Normal Oral Histology*. Quintessence: Chicago, 2000)

Fig 1-13 Photomicrograph of cementum positioned apical to the CEJ (5-10% of cases). (From Riviere, *Lab Manual of Normal Oral Histology*. Quintessence: Chicago, 2000)

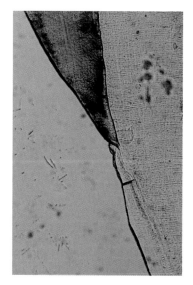

Fig 1-14 Photomicrograph of cementum positioned coronal to the CEJ, onto the enamel surface (60-65% of cases). (From Riviere, *Lab Manual of Normal Oral Histology*. Quintessence: Chicago, 2000)

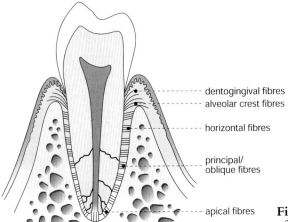

dentogingival fibres
alveolar crest fibres

horizontal fibres

principal/
oblique fibres

apical fibres

Fig 1-15 Schematic diagram of PDL.

- periodontal ligament fibres
  - alevolar crest fibres
  - horizontal fibres
  - principal/oblique fibres
  - apical fibres
- neurovascular channels
  - sensory fibres (pain, pressure and proprioception)
  - proprioreceptive fibres
  - autonomic fibres
  - blood vessels
  - lymphatics
- cellular elements
  - fibroblasts
  - cementoblasts/clasts
  - osteoblasts/clasts
  - undifferentiated mesenchymal cells (cells which under different stimuli can differentiate into any of the cells normally found within the PDL)
- ground substance.

The fibres of the PDL (Fig 1-15) protect the tooth from excessive forces by acting in a hydraulic environment, where tissue fluid lies between major fibre bundles and tooth displacement stimulates sensory and proprio-receptive (positional awareness) nerve conduction. The rate of fibre turnover is

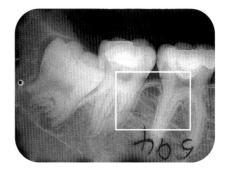

Fig 1-16 Radiograph showing healthy interdental crest with intact lamina dura and early demineralisation around adjacent tooth.

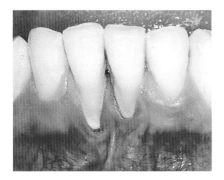

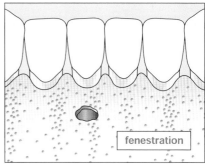

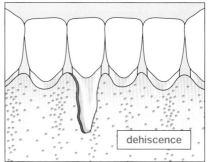

Fig 1-17 Schematic diagram of bony fenestration and dehiscences with clinical picture of Stillman's cleft above.

high and the fibroblasts are active. Naturally the tooth can move within the socket by a small degree and this is termed "*physiological mobility*" (up to 0.2mm).

Alveolar bone

The extended part of the mandible and maxilla that forms the tooth socket is called *alveolar bone* or the *alveolar process*. It is fine at its margin, becoming

15

thicker towards the root apex, and has dense facial and lingual cortical plates, which meet at the *alveolar crest*. The latter is situated 1–1.5mm apical to the CEJ in health and radiographically forms a point (Fig 1-16), unless the teeth are widely spaced, when a more rounded crest may form. In health, the cortical plate forms a continuous line linking one socket via the interdental crest to adjacent sockets, visible as a fine dense white line radiographically called the *lamina dura*. The first sign of bone demineralisation radio- graphically is the loss of the lamina dura, which often occurs first at the interdental alveolar crest. Vascular, lymphatic and neural channels from the cancellous bone beneath perforate the cortical plate of the tooth socket, supplying the PDL. The thickness of the cortical bone varies across the maxilla and mandible, being thinnest overlying the lower incisors and thickest overlying the mandibular molars. Developmental defects can arise most commonly over lower incisors, where bone is absent as a "window" called a *fenestration*, or the fenestration communicates with the alveolar margin forming a *dehiscence*. The absence of periosteum, which carries part of the gingival blood supply, in these areas, can make them prone to gingival recession and cleft formation, following repeated episodes of inflammation. Such soft tissue clefts are called *Stillman's* clefts (Fig 1-17).

Further Reading

Holmstrup, P. The Macroanatomy of the periodontium. In Wilson Jr TG, Kornman KS (Eds.) Fundamentals of Periodontics. Chicago: Quintessence, 1996: 17–45.

Chapter 2
How Does Plaque Cause Disease?

Aim

The concept that plaque causes gingivitis is a fact, proven by a series of studies in the 1960s. Whether plaque causes periodontitis is a different debate. Without plaque bacteria, inflammatory periodontitis would not occur, but in the presence of plaque bacteria, periodontitis often does not occur. This chapter aims to explain the mechanisms by which periodontal microorganisms may cause disease in a susceptible host, given the right circumstances.

Outcome

The outcome of reading this chapter will be that the reader will understand the microbial basis for contemporary and future periodontal therapies. The reader will also appreciate the complexities of a poly-microbial infection, as opposed to mono-infections like HIV or TB, and why the use of systemic antibiotics in periodontal management is of limited benefit for all but a limited number of patients.

A Model for Periodontal Disease Pathogenesis

Whether periodontitis develops in an individual depends upon a myriad of complex issues collectively called "risk factors" (see Chapter 4). Unlike gingivitis, which develops in the majority of, if not all, humans, periodontitis is multi-factorial and cannot be regarded as a pure infection like HIV disease or TB. It is polymicrobial (Fig 2-1) and there are many "*host factors*" (see Chapter 3), some genetically determined and some environmentally determined, which impact on the following clinical issues:

- Will periodontal disease develop in this patient?
- If so, at what age will it develop?
- What type of disease will develop? ("classification" – see Chapter 6)
- At what rate will the disease progress?
- What pattern of disease progression should we look for? (see Chapter 5)
- How will this patient respond to therapy?
- What is the most appropriate therapy for this case?

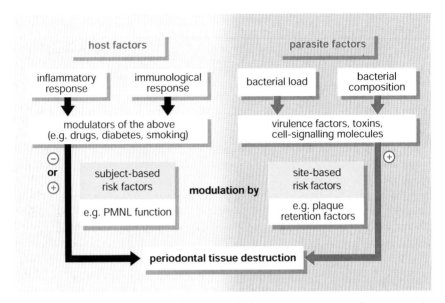

Fig 2-1 Schematic diagram showing how a delicate balance can exist between periodontal bacteria and the host. Tissue damage can result from bacteria overpowering the immune response or from products of the host's own inflammatory–immune response, if this is exaggerated. On top of this are a large number of modifying or risk factors which can exist at the individual patient or systemic level, or at the individual periodontal site level (Chapter 4).

- Will teeth be lost? And if so, how many?
- May there be systemic consequences of the disease process or its treatment?

Without bacteria there would be no periodontal disease, but bacteria are essential to maintain health and of the 700-plus species already known to exist in the oral cavity (some 400–500 colonising the periodontal tissues), only a few cause disease.

A "pathogen" is an organism that causes disease.
A "commensal" is a non-disease-forming organism; part of the resident flora.
"Opportunist pathogens" are normally not pathogenic, but are able to become so if their local environment is changed (e.g. by antibiotic therapy eliminating competing bacteria, or in an immunocompromised host). They can overgrow and the "microbial load" that results can cause disease.

How Do Bacteria Cause Disease?

Bacteria normally cause disease when the following basic sequences occur:
- acquisition
- adherence or retention
- initial survival
- prosperity and longer-term survival
- avoidance of elimination
- multiplication
- elaboration of "virulence factors".

Acquisition of oral bacteria occurs at birth from parental (called *vertical transmission*) and other environmental sources. This has led to the concept of *endogenous organisms* (already present in the host when the disease develops) and *exogenous organisms* (those acquired from other individuals or the environment, which may initiate the disease process or enable its progression). In 1993, Van Steenbergen and colleagues used genetic fingerprinting methods to demonstrate that periodontal pathogens like *Actinobacillus actinomycetemcomitans* (*Aa*) and *Porphyromonas gingivalis* (*Pg*) can be transmitted between individuals within families. In one study in 1988 by Preus and Olsen, transmission between an adolescent and the family dog was demonstrated. However, in chronic periodontitis it is likely that causative organisms are endogenous. If exogenous sources become involved, chronic exposure is necessary for colonisation of the new host. Whilst periodontal disease is not thought to be transmitted by kissing, it is worth remembering that repeated failure of periodontal therapy in an individual may be due to re-infection from chronic contact with a partner.

Adherence/retention describes the ability of an organism to attach to a surface, and is essential for bacterial survival unless the bacteria are planktonic (able to swim and survive in a dynamic manner). It is for this reason that the eruption of teeth in mammals provides a non-shedding, stable surface for organisms to adhere to. The first organisms to adhere to the glycoprotein pellicle that forms on crown surfaces within minutes of removal are called "pioneer" organisms. Gram-positive cocci like "streptococci" have this ability via production of mucopolysaccharides, and gram-negative organisms possess cell wall components called lipoteichoic acids, which facilitate adhesion. Such mechanisms also assist the retention of organisms in environments where physical adhesion is not an absolute requirement for colonisation, e.g. habitats not exposed to physical forces such as salivary flow.

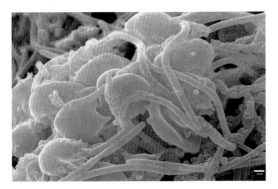

Fig 2-2 A scanning electron micrograph (SEM) of a microbial biofilm demonstrating the intimate relationship of motile organisms with static organisms. Rod-shaped organisms can be seen along with cocci, filamantous bacteria and spirochaetes and blood cells from the host.

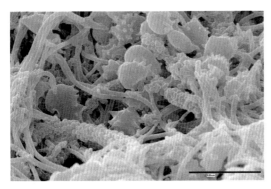

Fig 2-3 SEM showing intimate relationship of bacteria within a biofilm. The alignment of cocci along the length of a filament is called a "corn-on-the-cob" relationship.

Initial survival of an organism not only requires adhesion to a static surface, but also requires the acquisition of essential nutrients. The production of an extracellular matrix (comprising dextrans and levans) facilitates attachment to the tooth surface. Additionally, plaque adhering at the gingival margin and interproximally is more resistant to physical removal by the forces of the oral musculature, food particles and washing by saliva. Within the gingival crevice, GCF is rich in all serum components, including glucose (raised in GCF in hyperglycaemic individuals) and iron. The crevice is, nevertheless, a hostile environment since GCF also contains iron-binding proteins like transferrin, haptoglobin and haemoglobin, as well as antibody and complement.

Prosperity and longer-term survival within the gingival crevice requires the bacteria to be able to survive relatively harmoniously with their neighbours in a "biofilm". A biofilm is a complex structure within which there are areas of high and low bacterial mass, interlaced with aqueous channels. Biofilms (Fig 2-2) function like multicellular organisms characterised by

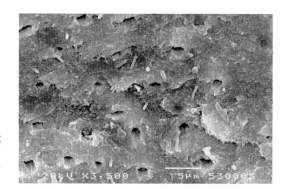

Fig 2-4 SEM demonstrating periodontal bacteria at the entrance of dentine tubules on the root surface.

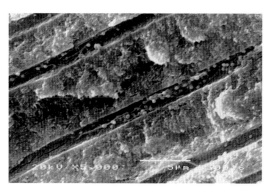

Fig 2-5 SEM showing bacteria within dentinal tubules with extra-cellular polysaccharide matrix production.

shedding of bacterial surface components (e.g. antigens, which can activate a host immune response) and release of various toxins (e.g. endotoxin, which activates a host inflammatory response). Within this environment, bacteria are capable of an activity called *"quorum sensing"*, which is simply being able to respond to products or signals from other biofilm organisms, or the host, and to use these to grow and prosper; some organisms physically adhere to each other (Fig 2-3).

Avoidance of elimination by the host defence system is a key strategy of all pathogens. Bacterial capsules can facilitate this and some organisms undergo genetic *"shift and drift"* whereby certain surface antigens mutate such that host antibodies can no longer recognise and bind to them. *Aa* produces:

- *leucotoxin* (an exotoxin) that destroys polymorphonuclear leucocytes (PMNLs or neutrophils)
- *epitheliotoxin*
- *immunoglobulin proteases* (factors capable of breaking down antibody).

21

Pg also produces a battery of proteases called "gingipains", which can damage antibody, complement, and other connective tissue components. Some organisms are able to sequestrate themselves within dentine tubules, providing a pool for re-colonisation of periodontal pockets, post-root surface debridement (Fig 2-4). The use of antibiotics is counter-productive in chronic periodontitis, because by the time the active agent has penetrated the biofilm, its concentration is too low to be effective and resistant strains of bacteria can emerge. Systemic antibiotics should only be contemplated in conjunction with mechanical debridement in aggressive forms of periodontitis. Biofilm organisms are 500-fold more resistant to antimicrobial strategies than organisms that do not occupy biofilms, because the extracellular matrix slows down diffusion of host defence products and forms a reservoir of microbial products which can inhibit host defences.

Multiplication is essential for longer-term survival and periodontal pathogens need to reach a certain critical mass within the subgingival biofilm to survive. Even once this critical mass is achieved, it is believed that further multiplication beyond a certain "threshold" is necessary for disease induction. What tips the balance for such pathogens beyond this threshold is uncertain: it may be a transient suppression of the immune system by stress, medication or other infections (e.g. HIV), or the ability of such organisms to respond to host-derived chemicals or hormones. One possible mechanism for this is under investigation in our own laboratories and those of collaborators, and has shown that certain periodontal organisms may use noradrenaline (produced during stress responses) to produce an "*auto-inducer*". The latter stimulates their own growth and that of other organisms found within the hostile environment of the periodontal pocket, potentially enabling shifts in biofilm composition to occur in response to changes in the local host environment.

Elaboration of "virulence factors" is essential for the production of disease. The "virulence" of an organism describes its *power* to produce disease. Broadly there are three categories of virulence factors:
- *Enzymes* (e.g. collagenase, hyaluronidase, elastase, anti-complement enzymes, those that break antibody down and many others). Such enzymes are believed to be able to break down the epithelial inter-cellular cement (called cadherin molecules), allowing entry into the connective tissues, where they can cause more damage than is possible within the "external" gingival crevice.
- *Metabolic waste products* such as ammonia, volatile fatty acids, cytotoxic amines and hydrogen sulphide (H_2S). Some periodontal pathogens have

been shown to metabolise protective anti-inflammatory and antioxidant peptides like glutathione to form toxic compounds like H_2S.

- *Toxins* which are either *endotoxins* or *exotoxins*
  - *Endotoxins* – so called, because they are only released from the cell walls of gram-negative bacteria largely when they die, but slow release can also occur within vesicles or through soluble forms. Also known as lipopolysaccharide (LPS), these are among the most potent stimulators of immune and inflammatory responses and subsequent host tissue damage. They attach loosely to cementum and are easily washed away by the irrigant from ultrasonic or sonic scalers. Other properties of endotoxins include:
    - Loose association with the top 10–15% of cementum.
    - Activation of clotting factors (e.g. Hageman factor) causing intravascular coagulation, thrombosis and ischaemic necrosis of areas of the gingiva.
    - Complement activation (see Chapter 3) and subsequent inflammation.
    - Priming of phagocytes in preparation for "activation" and release of enzymes and oxygen radicals.
    - Activation of the immune response (antigenicity).
    - Macrophage toxicity.
    - Bone resorption (e.g. *Aa* and *Pg*).
    - Fibroblast toxicity.
    - Inhibition of connective tissue attachment (collagen).
  - *Exotoxins* – are released by living bacteria and include the leucotoxin of *Aa* and others previously mentioned.

Maturation of the Plaque Biofilm

S. sanguis (a gram-positive *streptococcus*) is one of the first organisms to colonise the crown surface at 24 hours, followed by gram-positive rods and filamentous bacteria of the *Actinomyces* species. Such organisms are not strictly *aerobic* (requiring oxygen to survive) or *anaerobic* (unable to survive in oxygen), but are known as *facultative* organisms (can survive with or without oxygen). As plaque matures during the development of gingivitis and the subgingival biofilm develops, the flora shifts towards a gram-negative rather than a gram-positive flora, and becomes more *motile* (greater numbers of planktonic organisms) and anaerobic. The pocket flora is largely anaerobic, gram-negative and heavily motile, with spirochaetes populating the biofilm base.

Microbial Invasion

To cause tissue damage, bacteria or their products must enter the periodontal tissues. Whether periodontal bacteria physically invade host tissue *in vivo* or not is controversial, with the exception of *necrotising ulcerative gingivitis (NUG)* and *periodontitis (NUP)* (see Chapter 6), where, in 1965. Listgarten and co-workers demonstrated invasion. Once micro-ulcers form within the SE (see Chapter 1), bacteria will colonise such sites. However, whether they directly cause the ulceration through release of enzymes, or whether it results from the host's inflammatory response (via enzymes and oxygen radicals released from phagocytes as they pass across the JE), or a combination of both (most likely), is unclear. *In vitro* invasion has been demonstrated for a number of pathogens including *Pg* and *Bacteroides forsythus (Bf)*. *In vivo* invasion is, however, harder to study, and whilst *Bf* has been demonstrated by Dibart and colleagues (1998) inside epithelial cells (see Fig 7a,b), the organisms were seen inside vacuoles and are most likely to have been pinocytosed by the epithelial cells.

Which Organisms Cause Periodontal Diseases?

A number of hypotheses have emerged over the years in an attempt to explain how bacteria cause periodontal diseases.

The specific plaque hypothesis
In 1976, Loesche proposed that specific microorganisms were necessary for the development of periodontal disease, i.e. it is the quality of bacteria rather than the quantity that matters. There is good evidence to link *Aa* to localised aggressive periodontitis and *Pg* to generalised aggressive periodontitis, but both organisms are found in non-diseased sites and may also be absent when the respective diseases are present clinically. There are many reasons for this, but the most likely explanation is that *Aa* and other putative pathogens have several "*clonal types*", and only a minority are virulent. This places limitations on microbial testing and identification in the diagnosis of periodontal diseases, as all but the most complex tests are not specific to sub-species clones. The majority of these putative pathogens exist deep within the pocket in anaerobic conditions and are highly susceptible to environmental change (fragile), induced by physical instrumentation.

The non-specific plaque hypothesis
In 1986, Thielade proposed that the disease results from the shear mass of organisms present and once this exceeds a certain threshold, disease will

occur. In 1965, Löe and co-workers performed a series of "experimental gingivitis" studies which taken together proved that plaque-induced gingivitis fitted the non-specific model. Plaque was allowed to accumulate around the teeth of dental students for 21 days and mild gingivitis resulted. However, plaque accumulates more readily around the margins of gingivae that are inflamed than around un-inflamed tissues, so, to prove "cause and effect", the plaque had to be removed leading to subsequent resolution of the gingivitis. Even then, some argued that it was the lack of stimulation of gingival blood flow by brushing that may have caused the inflammation, rather than the build up of plaque, so the study had to be repeated using the antiseptic chlorhexidine, rather than brushing, finally to prove the relationship.

The environmental plaque hypothesis

Described by Haffajee and colleagues in 1991, the environmental plaque hypothesis suggests the entire subgingival microbial environment is the key to disease developing. Eliminating commensal species like *S sanguis* (*Ss*) from a periodontal site may also result in the elimination of true pathogens which depend upon *Ss* for certain nutrients. In chronic periodontitis, of the between 300 and 500 species which colonise the pocket, only 10–30 are thought to be pathogenic. Therefore, to develop periodontitis, not only is a susceptible host necessary, but pathogenic species must emerge in sufficiently high numbers from within the subgingival biofilm. Current evidence would support this hypothesis as the most appropriate for chronic periodontitis.

Stratification of Organisms Within the Pocket and Cluster Analysis

A group in Boston, Massachusetts lead by Socransky, has investigated over many years the periodontal microflora in health and disease (Table 2-1) and how periodontal bacteria change along the length of a periodontal pocket. Most recently, work analysing large numbers of species from individual periodontal pockets has demonstrated that certain organisms cluster together, in discrete micro-environments. These complexes have been colour coded as:

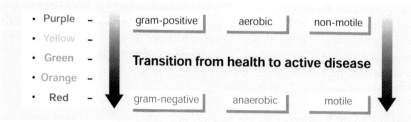

Table 2-1 **Periodontal microorganisms and associated conditions**

Condition	Organism
Gingival health	*Streptococcus sanguis* *Actinomyces viscosus* *Streptococcus oralis*
Necrotising ulcerative gingivitis	*Treponema vincentii* *Fusobacterium nucleatum* *Prevotella intermedia* *Candida species ?*
Gingivitis	*Fusobacterium nucleatum* *Porphyromonas gingivalis*
Localised aggressive periodontitis	*Actinobacillus actinomycetemcomitans*
Generalised aggressive periodontitis	*Porphyromonas gingivalis*
Chronic periodontitis	*Porphyromonas gingivalis* *Bacteroides forsythus* *Fusobacterium nucleatum* *Campylobacter recta* *Eikonella corrodens* *Peptostreptococcus micros* *Prevotella intermedia* *Eubacterium species* *Spirochaete species*

Haffajee listed the properties a bacterium must posses to cause periodontitis:
- It must be of a virulent clonal type.
- It must posses the genetic chromosomal factors to initiate the disease.
- The host must be susceptible to the pathogen.
- The numbers of pathogens within a clone must exceed a threshold for that host.
- It must be located at the correct site.

Table 2-2 **Socransky's mocrobial complexes**

Complex	Clustering organisms
Purple (gram-positive rods and cocci)	*Veillonella parvula* *Actinomyces odontolyticus I*
Yellow (gram-positive facultative cocci)	*Streptococcus sanguis* *Streptococcus gordonii* *Streptococcus intermedius* *Streptococcus oralis* *Streptococcus mitis*

Green
(gram-positive and gram-negative rods/cocci – non-motile)
	Eikenella corrodens
	Actinobacillus actinomycetmecomitans
	    serotype a
	Capnocytophagia ochracea
	Capnocytophagia sputigena
	Capnocytophagia gingivalis
	Actinobacillus actinomycetmecomitans
	    serotype b

Orange (gram-positive and negative rods/cocci – some motility)	*Fusobacterium nucleatum ssp. polymorphum* *Fusobacterium nucleatum ssp. nucleatum* *Prevotella intermedia* *Streptococcus constellatus* *Eubacterium nodatum* *Campylobacter gracilis* *Camylobacter rectus* *Peptostreptococcus micros* *Prevotella nigescens* *Fusobacterium periodonticum* *Fusobacterium nucleatum ssp. vincentii* *Campylobacter showae*
Red (gram-negative, anaerobic and motility)	*Porphyromonas gingivalis* *Bacteroides forsythus* *Treponema denticola*

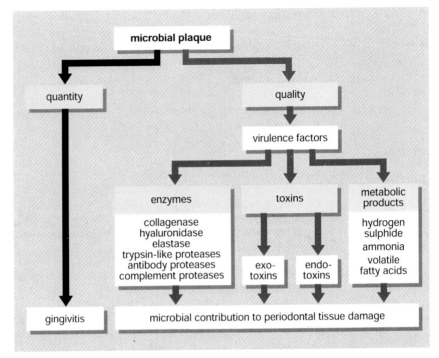

Fig 2-6 Schematic representation of how periodontal micro-organisms may cause tissue damage.

- Other species must support or at least not inhibit the pathogen.
- The local environment must be conducive to the production of virulence factors.

Fig 2-6 summarises the role of periodontal bacteria in disease pathogenesis.

Conclusions of Clinical Importance

- Gingivitis is a disease caused by the progressive accumulation of plaque at the gingival margin – plaque removal results in resolution.
- The majority of patients may suffer from gingivitis.
- Specific bacteria cause chronic periodontitis, but these exist in a subgingival biofilm, where self-support and protection provide resistance to elimination.
- Only a small number of patients (5%–15%) appear susceptible to periodontitis.

- Antibiotics are not normally indicated in the management of chronic periodontitis.
- Physical disruption of the biofilm is essential to eliminate fragile anaerobic pathogens.
- Pathogens in chronic periodontitis are likely to be endogenous to the host.
- Pathogens can be transmitted within families.
- Failure of therapy may be due to factors peculiar to the patient, but may also be due to re-infection from a partner or family member.
- Recurrence of disease may be due to viral organisms.

Further Reading

Dibart S, Skobe Z, Snapp KR, Socransky SS, Smith CM, Kent R. Identification of bacterial species on or in crevicular epithelial cells from healthy and periodontally diseased patients using DNA-DNA hybridization. Oral Microbiol Immunol 1998;13:30-35.

Haffajee AD, Socransky SS, Smith C, Dibart S. Microbial risk indicators for periodontal attachment loss. J Periodont Res 1991;26:293-296.

Löe H, Theilade E, Jensen SB. Experimental gingivitis in man. J Periodontol 1965;35:177-187.

Loesche WJ. Chemotherapy of dental plaque infections. Oral Sci Rev 1976;9:65-107.

Preus HR, Olsen I. Possible transmittance of *A. actinomycetemcomitans* from a dog to a child with rapidly destructive periodontitis. J Periodont Res 1988;23:68-71.

Socransky SS, Haffajec AD, Cugini MA, Smith C, Kent RL Jr. Microbial complexes in sub-gingival plaque. J Clin Periodontol 1998;25:134-144.

Theilade E. The non-specific theory in microbial aetiology of inflammatory periodontal disease. J Clin Periodontol 1986;13:905-911.

Van Steenbergen TJM, Petit MD, Scholte LH, van der Velden U, de Graaff J. Transmission of *porphyromonas gingivalis* between spouses. J Clin Periodontol 1993;20:340-345.

Chapter 3
The Role of the Host Response

Aim

No text in periodontology can avoid discussing the inflammatory and immune responses: subjects which confuse and thus bore many practitioners, often appearing to have little practical utility in the dental surgery. This chapter is the most complex in the book, but attempts to provide a substantially visual guide to key processes that govern disease development and hence therapeutic strategies. The chapter is essential to understanding the remainder of the text, and whilst contemporary, it must also prepare readers for new diagnostic and treatment strategies, some of which are already in the high street.

Outcome

The outcome of reading this chapter will be that the previously mystical world of periodontal immunopathology will make some sense. The reader will also be able to make informed decisions about whether he/she feels certain newer diagnostic tests and therapeutic strategies, whilst biologically effective, are worthwhile, in financial and logistical terms, for their *individual* patient.

The host–response to microbial plaque is designed to be protective, but the balance is a delicate one where under–activity or indeed over–activity of specific aspects of the response can lead to tissue destruction (Fig 3-1). For example, the patient in Fig 3-2 suffers from the defective function of an enzyme called C1-esterase inhibitor. The enzyme inhibits the activation of complement component C1 (which propagates inflammatory processes). When plaque accumulates at the gingival margin in her mouth, the resulting inflammation and swelling are exaggerated and cause severe gingival oedema and bone loss. There are two main components of the host-response to plaque:
- natural or innate immunity
- acquired or specific immunity.

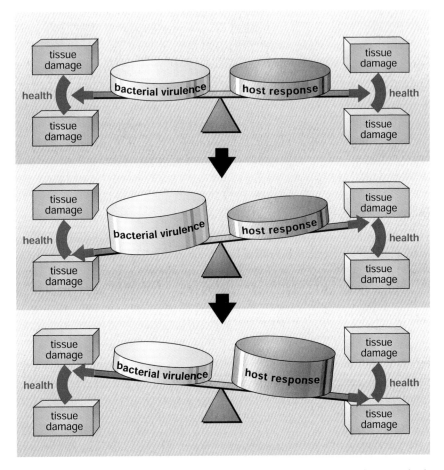

Fig 3-1 The delicate balance between parasitic activity and host defences, which maintain periodontal tissue health. Such equilibrium may easily be disrupted, leading to inflammation and tissue damage.

Both types of immunity are involved in the host's response to plaque and occur at the same time, but the innate system is constantly in function and more rapidly mobilisable, whereas the acquired system involves lymphocytes and specific cell–cell interactions which take more time. Early gingival inflammation largely involves the innate system, the acquired system becoming involved in moderate-to-advanced gingivitis and in periodontitis (i.e. longer-term, chronic disease).

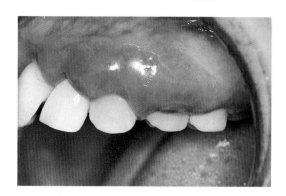

Fig 3-2 Clinical photograph of exaggerated inflammation in a patient with excellent oral hygiene, who suffers from C1-esterase inhibitor dysfunction.

Innate Immunity

This system is the first line of defence. Throughout evolution, it has been highly conserved, and, whilst rapid, it remains crudely indiscriminate relative to the specificity of the acquired system. In terms of periodontal immunology, it is akin to hitting a small nail with a sledgehammer, and hence, when something goes wrong with this system, the *collateral tissue damage* is significant. Innate immunity involves:

- intact epithelial barriers
- lubrication of epithelium with fluids (saliva, GCF) containing anti-bacterial factors
- the complement cascade
- cell-signalling molecules called *cytokines* (e.g. the interleukin family) and *chemokines* (molecules produced by one cell, which recruit specific leucocytes)
- vasoactive peptides (like histamine) released from mast cells
- adhesion molecules
- PMNL (neutrophil) defence systems
- macrophages – which also function as *antigen presenting cells* (APCs) at the beginning of specific immune responses.

Epithelial Barriers

Epithelial barriers were discussed in Chapter 1. The unique nature of the JE, its rapid rate of turnover and permeability to GCF and PMNLs passing through, provide primary first-line defence strategies. The epithelial cells also release cell-signalling molecules (see below) to help start the inflammatory process.

Fluid Lubrication

Whole, mixed saliva contains anti-bacterial enzymes, like lysozyme, and immunoglobulins (antibody) like IgA and IgG, which bind to bacteria. GCF carries all components of serum, including complement and immunoglobulin.

Complement Cascade

The complement cascade is a series of 20 serum glycoproteins, which circulate in inactive forms in the blood stream. When activated, complement components have profound and powerful effects in stimulating inflammation (pro-inflammatory effects). The main role of complement activation is:

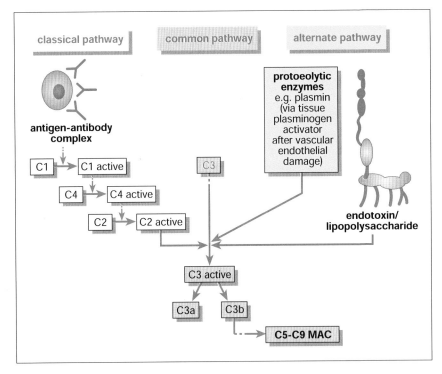

Fig 3-3 The complement cascade.

Table 3-1 **Some important effects of complement**

Complement Component	Inflammatory Effect
C3a and C5a	↑ blood vessel permeability via mast cell degranulation and release of histamine
C3b and C5a	Production of oxygen radicals by leucocytes
C5a	Leucocytes stick (marginate) to blood vessel walls Neutrophils release enzymes and oxygen radicals (called degranulation)
C3a	Chemotaxis of phagocytes (chemical attraction)
C3b	Cytokine (from lymphocytes) production Macrophage secretion Opsonisation (attraction and adhesion of phagocytes)
C5a and C567 complex	Leucocyte chemotaxis (movement towards infection)
C5b, C6, C7, C8 and C9	Lysis (splitting open) of gram-negative bacteria Host cell destruction

- recruitment of more phagocytes to the area of infection
- to facilitate binding of phagocytes (e.g. PMNLs) to bacteria, thereby aiding phagocytosis – a process called *opsonisation*
- to cause bacterial killing (cell lysis).

There are two pathways for complement activation (Fig 3-3):
- *alternative pathway* – activated directly by bacterial endotoxin (LPS) when it enters the periodontal tissues and from the cementum reservoir. Other proteolytic enzymes like plasmin and some neuropeptides (e.g. β-endorphin, released during stress responses) can also activate the alternative pathway.
- *classical pathway* – only activated by the formation of antigen-antibody complexes (i.e. after initiation of the acquired immune response).

Table 3-2 **Some important cytokines and their effects**

Cytokine	Cell of Origin	Effects Upon Inflammatory/ Immune Response
Interleukin 1 (**IL–1**)	macrophage (MØ), fibroblast, monocytes upon stimulation by endo/exotoxins epithelial cells	activation of osteoclasts ↑ PMNL margination ↑ prostaglandin PGE$_2$ by fibroblasts ↑ IL-6 synthesis by periodontal fibroblasts ↑ TNF-α production and release
Interleukin 6 (**IL–6**)	MØ, fibroblasts, epithelial cells	↑ acute phase protein synthesis by liver ↑ bone resorption ↑ B-cell differentiation and Ig production ↑ T-cell activation
Interleukin 8 (**IL–8**)	MØ, endo/epithelial cells LPS stimulated fibroblasts, platelets	potent PMNL chemotaxin
Interleukin 10 (**IL–10**)	T-lymphocytes B-lymphocytes	suppression of cytokines (anti-inflam-matory)
Transforming growth factor beta (TGF-β)	most cells	anti-inflammatory (at high concentrations) stimulates collagen synthesis and repair
Tumour necrosis factor alpha (TNF-α)	activated MØs monocytes epithelial cells	↑ MØ production of IL-1 ↑ MØ production of PGE-2 ↑ ICAM-1 expression / PMNL margina-tion ↑ PMNL oxygen radical production ↑ PMNL degranulation of enzymes
Prostaglandin E2 (PGE$_2$)	activated MØs monocytes PMNLs mast cells epithelial cells	↑ vascular permeability ↑ vasodilation ↑ PMNL-chemotaxis stimulates bone resorption
Granuloctye-macrophage colony stimulating factor (GM-CSF)	epithelial cells monocytes endothelial cells fibroblasts	↑ release of PMNLs from bone marrow ↑ PMNL chemotaxis ↓ apoptosis ↑ degranulation ↑ oxygen radical formation

Both pathways stimulate the activation of complement component C3, which leads to the activation of C5 and the amplification cascade which forms C5-C9, the so-called *membrane attack complex* (MAC). The methods by which active forms of C3 to C9 recruit phagocytes and propagate inflammation are summarised in Table 3-1. It can be seen how endotoxin can directly activate this cascade and, via complement component C3b, mediate the crude adherence of PMNLs to bacteria (opsonisation). PMNL-killing of the bacteria then follows through *extracellular* or *intracellular* killing mechanisms (see later), which may not involve lymphocytes and specific immunity. This type of action is believed to be responsible for early gingivitis.

Cell-signalling Molecules

Several families of these potent molecules exist; some stimulate cells to release other molecules (cytokines), some attract cells to areas of infection (chemokines) and others stimulate cells to perform other functions (cytokines and lymphokines). The function and dynamics of these highly complex networks are poorly understood and many have seemingly conflicting activities, whilst others have common activities. The main cytokines and their functions in periodontal inflammation are listed in Table 3-2. One of the most important cytokines in periodontal disease is interleukin-1 (IL-1), as it causes bone resorption and is powerfully pro-inflammatory. The genes that code for IL-1 have different forms (polymorphisms) and Kornman and colleagues found that patients who suffered from advanced chronic periodontal disease possessed a polymorphism of IL-1 that resulted in overproduction. A "periodontitis susceptibility test" (PST) has been developed from this work, which identifies from a finger-prick blood sample the presence of the "risk" polymorphism. However, patients' smoking habits confound the results, and there is no clear evidence that a PST-positive result will mean the patient concerned will develop periodontal disease. In addition, a study in the UK failed to demonstrate the same results as the United States study in a UK cohort.

Vasoactive Peptides

Vasoactive peptides, like histamine, play a crucial role in the development of inflammation. Histamine is released from mast cells upon stimulation (e.g. by complement C3a and C5a or PGE2) and causes *vasodilation* to bring more blood cells and plasma proteins (e.g. complement, antibody) to the area of infection. Vasodilation also slows down blood flow through vessels, allowing PMNLs to touch the vessel walls, rather than being carried mid-

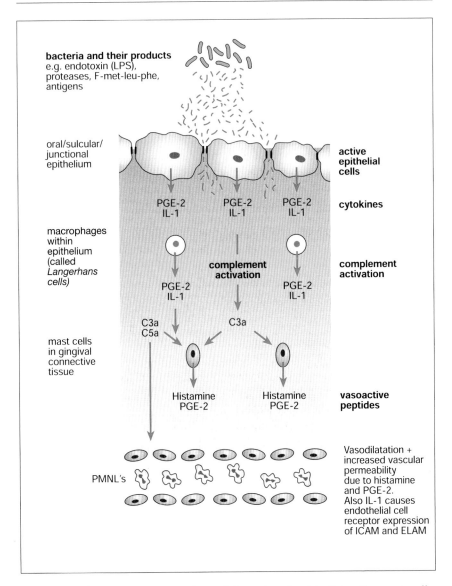

Fig 3-4 Schematic representation of the role of epithelial cells, mast cells, macrophages and complement in the production of cytokines and vasoactive peptides that produce key vascular changes in early inflammation.

stream within blood (see below). Histamine also increases *vascular permeability* to allow defence products within plasma to enter the tissues. The main phagocytes are neutrophils (PMNLs) and blood monocytes, which when they enter tissues become macrophages or Langerhans cells (epithelial macrophages). Fig 3-4 illustrates the role of cytokines and vasoactive peptides in the early vascular changes that enable inflammation to progress.

Adhesion Molecules

As the name suggests, adhesion molecules are used by host cells to stick to each other or to components of the intercellular matrix. Various terms are used to describe such molecules: for example, adhesion molecules, receptors (e.g. integrins or selectins), ligands, etc. The key concept to grasp when attempting to understand innate immunity is that cellular trafficking into and within the tissues is not a random process: it is directed by signalling molecules and adhesion molecules in very specific sequences and pathways. Examples of important adhesion molecules are intercellular adhesion molecules I and II (ICAM-I and II), endothelial adhesion molecule 1 (ELAM-I) and leucocyte function antigen-1 (LFA-1). These molecules may or may not be expressed on a cell surface, and expression can be turned on or off by cytokines (e.g. IL-1, IL-10). Fig 3-5 illustrates the role of cytokines in the expression of adhesion molecules and how these stick to PMNL receptors to cause the following sequence of events:

- *Rolling* – slowing down of PMNLs within the blood stream occurs due to vasodilation, following the release of vasoactive peptides. "Make and break" contacts between PMNL receptors (called *selectins*) and complementary ones on vascular endothelial cells are then able to occur.
- *Margination* – as the PMNL slows down the receptor binding becomes stronger and the PMNL becomes immobilised on the vascular endothelium by adhesion of *integrin* molecules (e.g. LFA-1) with complementary endothelial receptors (e.g. ICAM-I)
- *Diapedesis* – Other cell-to-cell adhesions allow the PMNL to pass through the "leaky" vessel wall (leaky due to histamine, etc.) and enter the tissues.
- *Chemotaxis* – The PMNL now moves along a chemical gradient, attracted by chemotaxins, which may be of bacterial or host origin.

The Polymorphonuclear Leucocyte (or Neutrophil/PMNL)

The PMNL is the most abundant and important defence cell in the periodontal tissues. Even in clinical health, PMNLs are found passing out of blood vessels within the gingiva, and through the connective tissues into the

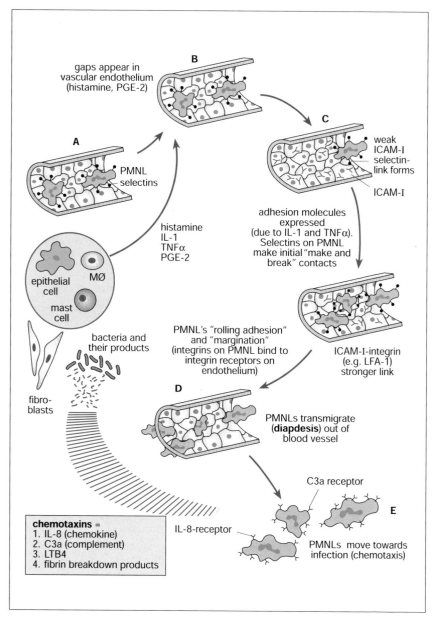

Fig 3-5 Schematic representation of the processes involved in the recruitment of neutrophils from blood vessels to sites of tissue damage and infection.

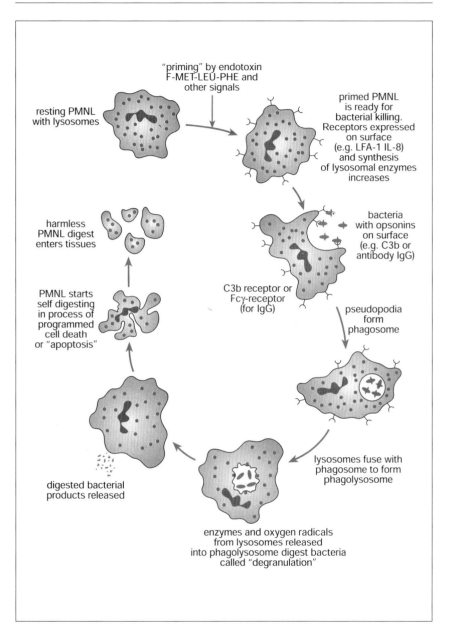

Fig 3-6 Schematic representation of the processes involved in neutrophil killing by intracellular mechanisms.

gingival crevice and ultimately saliva. Neutrophils have a short life-expectancy of only 24 hours and have four main components of functional importance:

- *Receptors* – on the PMNL surface respond to many different stimuli. Some help it to bind to the vessel wall (e.g. integrins like LFA-1); or recognise chemical attractants (e.g. receptors for chemotaxins like C3a or IL-8); others help it stick to bacteria through opsonisation (e.g. receptors for complement C3b or antibody receptors called Fc-receptors).

- *Cytoskeleton* – Clearly, in order to move, the PMNL has within it an internal skeleton made of actin muscle fibres (*actin cytoskeleton*).

- *Lysosomes* – are also called neutrophil *granules*. There are primary, secondary and non-specific granules, which essentially contain the enzymes used to destroy bacterial structures (e.g. PMNL elastase, cathepsins, phosphatases, collagenases, lipases, etc.)

- *Oxygen Radicals* – The PMNL contains a special "shunt" called the NADPH-oxidase or hexose-monophosphate shunt. This is situated on the inner PMNL-cell membrane and simply shunts hexose and NADPH out of the energy- (ATP-) producing cycle, and uses them to reduce oxygen to form oxygen radicals (the so-called *respiratory burst*). These include *superoxide* and related species like *hydrogen peroxide* and *hydroxyl radicals,* which destroy bacterial (and host) tissues.

Once the PMNL arrives at the site of infection, it kills bacteria by either *intracellular* or *extracellular* methods. Intracellular killing involves exactly the same methods as extracellular killing, except the PMNL releases its enzymes and oxygen radicals (a process called *degranulation*) safely within itself and inside special membrane-bound structures (see Fig 3-6). Clearly, the enzymes and oxygen radicals may also damage host tissue as well as bacterial tissue and the PMNL therefore contains:

- *enzyme inhibitors* – the main one being α-1 antitrypsin (neutralises enzymes like elastase)

- *antioxidants* – these are powerful scavengers of oxygen radicals (e.g. glutathione) and also involve enzyme systems (e.g. superoxide dismutase and catalase) to prevent damage to the PMNL during oxygen radical release.

Following intracellular killing of bacteria, the PMNL goes through a process of programmed cell death or *apoptosis*, whereby it essentially self-digests to prevent harmful contents entering the host tissues. Some pathogens like *Pg* produce anti-apoptosis factors believed to allow uncontrolled PMNL death and subsequently PMNL-mediated host tissue damage.

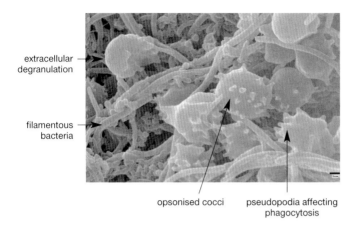

extracellular
degranulation

filamentous
bacteria

opsonised cocci   pseudopodia affecting
phagocytosis

Fig 3-7 SEM of a subgingival plaque sample, demonstrating cocci opsonised to PMNLs and active phagocytosis. Some PMNLs have degranulated extracellularly, due to the mass of bacteria being too large to engulf.

When the bacterial mass is too large for the PMNL to phagocytose (Fig 3-7), it degranulates extracellularly and releases its enzymes and oxygen radicals over the bacterial mass in an effort to cause as much damage as possible. If this occurs in the gingival crevice, it may damage crevicular epithelium, but where a massive PMNL response is present in the tissues, inadvertent release of these chemicals is believed to be the major cause of periodontal tissue damage and bone loss.

Macrophages (MØ)

Macrophages are scavengers of dead cells (bacterial or PMNLs), but also play an important role in bridging the gap between *innate immunity* and *acquired immunity*. As phagocytes, they function in a similar manner to PMNLs, but they also act as *antigen presenting cells* (APCs). Macrophages possess the same surface glycoproteins as all other human cells (except red blood cells) called MHC-antigens (MHC = major histocompatability complex; also called HLA or Human Leucocyte Antigens). There are two main types of MHC-antigens (class I and class II) and MHC-class II is the antigen system that enables the host's immune system to recognise "host" from "foreign" tissue. When macrophages come across cells they do not recognise, they phagocytose them and release onto their surface antigenic material from those cells that is linked to MHC-class II molecules. T-lymphocytes, already specific to the foreign material, recognise this complex of MHC-class II/foreign antigen, bind to it and then go on to mount a specific immune response. At the same time as *antigen presentation* to T-cells, the MØ releases IL-1 and TNF-α, which have the vascular effects described previously (Fig 3-4). Hence, the MØ has a role in innate immunity and also in stimulating acquired/specific immunity. MØs produce PGE_2, which causes bone resorption. Offenbacher and colleagues have found that monocytes (blood MØs) collected from peripheral blood of periodontitis patients produce considerably more PGE_2 than those from healthy controls, when given the same stimulus. Whether this is because the MØs in the diseased group were already *"primed"* by blood-borne endotoxin or whether disease-susceptible subjects produce inherently more PGE_2 is unknown.

Acquired/Specific Immunity

This final section will provide a brief overview of acquired immunity. It is important to remember that the innate immune response is occurring at the same time as the acquired response, but is less specific and thus less efficient. The acquired response involves:

− *T-lymphocytes*
− *B-lymphocytes*
− *Immunoglobulins.*

T-lymphocytes make up the *cell-mediated* immune response, so-called because the antigen-specific molecule on the T-cell (the T-cell receptor [TCR]) is not secreted/released from the cell, but remains stuck to the T-cell surface. Thus, direct contact between the T-cell and bacteria is necessary to cause bacterial destruction, i.e. the response is "mediated" by the T-cell itself and not by free antibody within serum.

B-lymphocytes form the *humoral immune* response, so-called because B-cells produce antigen-specific molecules (immunoglobulins – Igs). When this occurs they become plasma cells. The antigen-specific molecules are released from the plasma cell and enter tissue fluid (humor) and blood. Igs, with the help of complement and phagocytes, cause destruction of bacteria to which they are specific.

Immunoglobulins – There are five main classes, called IgG, IgA, IgM, IgD, IgE *(antibody/Igs)*. The most important in periodontal disease are IgG (from GCF) and IgA (from saliva).

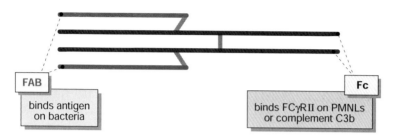

Fig 3-8 The structure of immunoglobulin.

Immunoglobulins

The first immunoglobulin to be produced in any infection is IgM, because it has five immunoglobulin units (i.e. it is a pentomer) and cross-links molecules well. IgG is produced later and is probably the most important antibody type, owing to its small molecular weight (monomeric) and ubiquity. IgG enters the gingival crevice and subsequently saliva from blood plasma, via GCF. Salivary immunoglobulin is of the IgA type, which is released as a dimer and emerges within saliva following the addition of a secretory unit (called a "J-chain!") by the gland. The basic structure of monomeric immunoglobulins is shown in Fig 3-8. There are four chains to the molecule, two *light chains* at the end that binds antigen (FAB [fragment that is antigen binding]), and two *heavy chains* running from the FAB end to the end that binds PMNL-receptors (Fc [fragment that is constant]). IgM and IgG activate (fix) complement; however, four types of IgG exist, called IgG1, IgG2, IgG3 and IgG4. IgG2 is poor at fixing complement and is therefore poor at bacterial killing and also a poor opsonin (see next paragraph).

The Fc parts of Igs differ in structure between classes and have different properties. The Fc of some antibodies is recognised by host defence cell receptors called Fc-receptors. The most common receptor on phagocytes is the Fcγ-receptor (Fcγ-R) of which there are several sub-types. Fcγ-RII is the PMNL-receptor thought to be most important for binding IgG2-opsonised bacteria. There are high and low avidity forms of Fcγ-RII, and in 1996, Wilson and Kalmar found that PMNL-receptors in black Americans who suffered from aggressive periodontitis had the form of Fcγ-RII that was of low avidity (i.e. did not bind IgG2 very well). This key discovery (see Chapter 4) has not been found in European patients suffering from aggressive periodontitis.

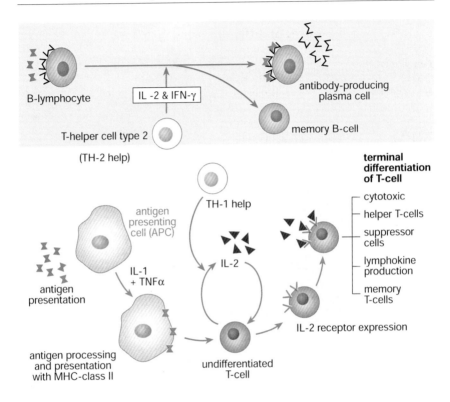

Fig 3-9 The cell-mediated and humoral immune responses.

T-Lymphocytes

The basic T-cell and B-cell immune processes are represented in Fig 3-9. It can be seen that cytokines like IL-1 and IL-2 play a major role in this process. Following presentation of processed antigen by APCs to the T-cell receptor, that un–differentiated T-cell expresses IL-2 receptor, which binds to IL-2 produced by T-helper cells (TH–1 cells) and causes terminal differentiation into effector T-cells.

T-lymphocytes differ from B-lymphocytes in a number of ways (see Table 3-3). The T-cells seem to be the first to arrive in the gingivitis lesion. Macrophages and Langerhans cells (APCs) carry antigen to the regional lymph nodes, and present this to undifferentiated T-cells. The T-cells commence transformation and homing signals initiate their trafficking back to

Table 3-3 **Some important differences between T-cells and B-cells**

Property	T-cell	B-cell
Receptor	TCR (T-cell receptor complex)	Immunoglobulin receptor (IgD or IgM)
Killing mechanism	Mediated by T-cell contact with target cell	Mediated by free immuno-globulin and phagocytes (i.e. B-cell not directly involved)
Killing capability	T-cell activity requires TH-1 help	B-cell activity requires TH-2 help
Sub-types	Several: T-cytotoxic T-suppressor T-helper Lymphokine production Memory cells	Fewer types: Plasma cells (active Ig secretors) Memory cells

the tissues. The homing signals are not yet understood, but cytotoxic T-cells reach the tissues and lyse bacteria in a specific manner. Memory T-cells remain within the lymph nodes and signalling molecules (lymphokines) from lymphokine producing T-cells attract macrophages, prevent their movement away from the infection and perform a variety of other functions including the assistance of B-cell function (T-helper type 2 cells – [TH-2 cells]). T-helper type 1 cells (TH-1) assist in T-cell functions.

B-Lymphocytes

B-lymphocytes largely require TH-2 cell help to produce antibody. Some B-cell activities can occur independently of TH-2 assistance, via T-cell in-dependent antigens. Importantly, endotoxin is an example of a T-cell independent antigen, capable of polyclonal B-cell activation, in the absence of TH-2 help. Binding of foreign antigen by immunoglobulin receptors on the B-cell surface largely occurs in the regional lymph nodes, but may also occur in the tissues. When stimulated, B-cells proliferate and then leave the lymph nodes and again "home" towards the tissues. In this manner, one stimulated B-cell can produce large numbers of clones to assist in host defence. When in the tissues, they enlarge due to the active protein synthesis occurring within to form plasma cells and produce immunoglobulin, which is released to bind to antigen. If plasma cell formation occurs in the lymph nodes, then immunoglobulin is released into the blood stream. The antigen-antibody complexes bind Fc receptors on PMNLs (opsonisation) and activate complement via the classical pathway. The Fc part of the Ig-bacterial complex also binds C3b, which again opsonises PMNLs. Plasma cells are too large to leave the lymph nodes and release antibody into the blood stream, from where it reaches the tissues. Plasma cells can form within the tissues, but appear at the late stages of periodontitis, when the immune response is well developed and are believed to be characteristic of an *active* periodontitis lesion. The *inactive* periodontitis lesion is characterised by T-lymphocytes, with fewer plasma-cells.

Conclusions of Clinical Importance

- In clinical health, PMNLs are the predominant defence cell, and innate immunity functions at a low level, without causing significant tissue damage.
- As plaque builds up, the actions of endotoxin, epitheliotoxin and others stimulate complement activation, which leads to a greater inflammatory response and gingival tissue damage.
- With time, the inflammatory lesion changes and T-lymphocytes appear, providing specific and controlled killing of bacterial cells.
- B-lymphocytes characterise an established lesion and freely produce antibody, which binds to antigen and activates the classical complement cascade.
- If left untreated in disease-susceptible patients, the size of the inflammatory response seems to exceed a threshold where host tissue damage occurs as a side-effect of the defence strategy.
- Active periodontal lesions are dominated by plasma cells, and the bulk of the tissue damage arises as "collateral" damage following release of enzymes and oxygen radicals by inflammatory cells.
- When the levels of enzymes and oxygen radicals exceed the host's enzyme-inhibitor and antioxidant defence strategies, connective tissue damage and bone loss occur.
- It is possible to modulate immune-inflammatory function in the treatment of periodontitis using anti-inflammatory drugs, but these do not reach into the tissues at significant levels. The key to therapy, therefore, remains the mechanical removal of the causative bacteria.

Further Reading

Host defences against microbial plaque. In Williams DM, Hughes FJ, Odell EW, Farthing PM. Pathology of Periodontal Disease. Oxford: Oxford Medical Publications, 1992: 67-96.

Kornman KS, Crane A, Wang HY, di Giovine FS, Newman MG, Pirk FW, Wilson TG, Higginbottom FL, Duff GW. The interleukin-1 genotype as a severity factor in adult periodontal disease. J Clin Periodontol 1997;24:72-77.

Galgutt PN, Dowsett SA, Kowolik MJ (Eds.) Periodontics: Current Concepts and Treatment Strategies. London: Martin Dunitz, 2001: 41-60.

Wilson ME, Kalmar JR. FcgRIIa (CD32): A potential marker defining susceptibility to localised juvenile periodontitis. J Periodontol 1996;67:323-331.

Chapter 4
Risk Assessment

Aim

Risk assessment has become a fundamental strategy employed when assessing any disease process and its subsequent management. This chapter aims to explain what *risk factors* are and how they differ from *risk markers* and *risk patients*. The most important risk factors for periodontitis will be discussed and a simple protocol outlined that will enable practitioners to account for risk factors in their periodontal patients, when formulating diagnoses, treatment plans and maintenance regimes.

Outcome

Having read this chapter the reader will appreciate the importance of the role of *risk factor analysis* in periodontal assessment and how such information informs diagnostic, treatment planning and maintenance strategies. It is hoped that the reader will also understand the key risk factors for periodontal disease and be able to implement a simple, rapid system of assessment within their daily practice.

Risk Assessment

Risk management is a term used in many working environments to describe the formalisation of a series of safety protocols that put common sense into practice. For example, the presence of a step at the threshold of a doorway leading from the waiting area to the surgery is likely to increase the risk of a patient tripping as they enter the surgery. Risk management would involve the practitioner identifying the risk during a formal risk assessment for their practice, and erecting a sign to draw patients' attention to it. Failure to do so could result in injury to a patient and a claim against the practice. The situation in periodontology is similar, since failure to identify proven risk factors for periodontitis results in failure to inform and educate the patient in fundamental issues relating to the disease process in their mouths. Furthermore, given that some risk factors can be modified or eliminated by the patient, e.g. smoking habit or level of diabetic control, practitioners have a duty of care to counsel patients appropriately about their role in the management

51

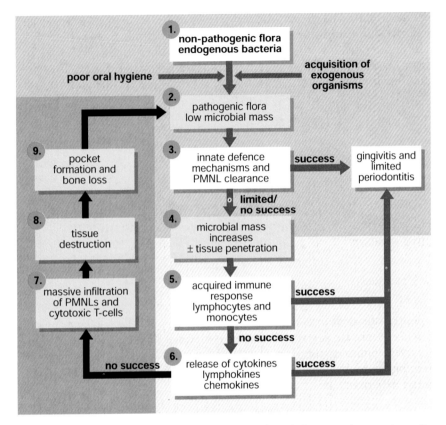

Fig 4-1 The "critical pathway model" for periodontal disease pathogenesis modified from Salvi *et al.* 1997.

of their periodontal disease. Management of periodontitis is a contract between the dental surgeon and the patient in which the successful outcome of therapy is dependent equally upon the patient doing "their bit" as it is on the dental team performing their duties to the highest possible standard.

Risk Factors

A risk factor is a factor that increases the probability that a disease may develop in an individual. Risk factors are biologically related to the occurrence of the disease, but they do not necessarily imply cause and effect: i.e. just because a patient possesses a risk factor does not mean that they will definitely develop the disease. Equally, absence of a risk factor does not mean that the disease will not develop. The majority of scientists advocate a two-stage model for disease development, in which a subject must possess genetic risk factors for a disease and then acquire environmental risk factors capable of exploiting that individual's inherent susceptibility to the disease. In periodontitis, risk factors are believed to modify the basic pathogenic process (Fig 4-1) and such risk factors result in a direct increase in the probability of acquiring the disease. They may be broadly categorised as:

1. *Systemic risk factors* (or "subject-based") – factors affecting one of the subject's "systems", which essentially affect the host-response to the plaque biofilm, upsetting the host-microbial balance (Fig 3-2).

2. *Local risk factors* (or "site-based") – factors local to the oral cavity, which may influence plaque accumulation or occlusal forces.

Risk Markers

Risk markers or predictors are not linked to "causation", but their presence is more a consequence of the disease being present. Risk markers imply the presence of disease and are often used to detect early stages of disease, before overt clinical signs become apparent. Examples would be the sign of bleeding on probing (BOP), tooth mobility, recession, suppuration, past disease experience, etc. (see Chapters 6 and 8).

Risk Patients

A risk patient is one who has a high probability of developing a disease over a specific period of time. Such patients either possess or have been exposed to "risk factors" for that disease. Therefore, a patient who smokes 30 cigarettes per day and has poor oral hygiene must be regarded as a risk patient for the development of periodontitis or necrotising ulcerative gingivitis (NUG) (see Chapter 6).

To help understand the role of risk factors, a model of disease pathogenesis that has been termed the "critical pathway model of pathogenesis" was developed by Offenbacher in 1996 (Fig 4-1). The model encompasses both the microbial and host components that contribute to periodontal destruction (Fig 2-1), but identifies nine key or critical stages in the process which must occur for disease development and progression. Each cycle of the closed loop represents further tissue destruction and risk factors may either lead to

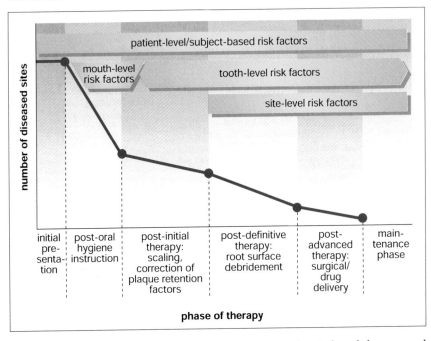

Fig 4-2 The potential effectiveness of different stages of periodontal therapy, and how levels of multiple risk assessment can apply to each stage.

PATIENT NAME:

REGISTRATION NO:

DATE OF BIRTH:

DIAGNOSIS: *Chronic moderate periodontitis*
(advanced disease UL67, UR 5, LL21 and LR12)

SYSTEMIC RISK FACTORS:

+ve family history ☐   Diabetes ☐
Smoker (pack years)_____   Stress ☐
Other _____

Fig 4-3 A simple tick-box system, which can be incorporated into an ink stamp and stamped in a susceptible patient's notes formally to record risk factors.

progress from one stage to the next within the loop, or to additional turns of the cycle. Equally, any critical stage may be reversed by successful host responses, or by elimination of risk factors.

Multi-Level Risk Assessment

One of the problems with risk assessment in periodontal disease is that the diseases are multifactorial and assessment should therefore be at multiple levels. The presence of pathogenic bacteria alone is not sufficient to cause the disease. In simple terms, there are four levels to consider:

1. The patient level	Perform at initial examination.
2. The whole mouth level	Perform at initial examination and post-initial therapy.
3. The tooth level	Perform post initial/definitive therapy and maintenance.
4. The site level	Perform post definitive therapy and during maintenance.

This approach also allows the clinician to separate risk factors that may initiate periodontal disease from those responsible for its progression or for the failure of initial therapy. A practical view to the application of the above is illustrated in Fig 4-2.

Patient-level risk assessment
Patient-level risk assessment can be determined at the initial consultation by performing the following:
- Family history (for hereditary/inborn/genetic risk factors). *"Is there a history of gum disease or pyorrhoea in the family – parents/grandparents – or early tooth loss?"*
- Medical history (for systemic diseases, e.g. diabetes).
- Present dental history (assess motivation to oral hygiene, etc.).
- Social history (smoking – current or former smoker).
- Habits (bruxism).

The majority of practitioners routinely collect such information, but its formal recording is recommended, perhaps alongside the diagnosis. For example, the use of a tick-box system with four key systemic risk factors would formalise this process (Fig 4-3).

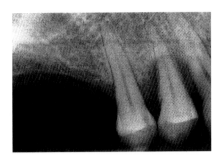

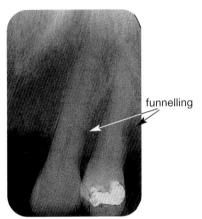

Fig 4-4 (a) A tooth subject to secondary occlusal trauma, as demonstrated by "crescentic" pattern of bone loss. In this situation, treatment of the periodontitis must take priority.

(b) A tooth subject to primary occlusal trauma demonstrates widening of the periodontal ligament space and early "funnelling". Elimination of the trauma will result in total bony resolution.

Mouth-level risk assessment
Mouth-level risk assessment would be performed at the initial examination, after a Basic Periodontal Examination (BPE) for susceptibility – as recommended by the British Society of Periodontology (Chapter 7) – and would include:

- Examination of attachment loss relative to age. This gives a very good idea of previous/current rates of progression and thus the likelihood of future rates of progression. It is important to remember that rapid progression of local lesions may still occur, despite a low age-related disease experience.
- Occlusal examination in static relationship (occlusal class, tooth wear, etc). A class 2 division II malocclusion with retroclined lower incisors can create hygiene problems for lingual surfaces of those teeth.
- Occlusal examination in dynamic relationship (patterns of guidance). Secondary occlusal trauma is trauma to a tooth that is already periodontally diseased, and can accelerate the disease process, but does not initiate it (Fig 4-4).
- Examination of levels of oral hygiene (Fig 4-5). A subject with periodontitis but excellent oral hygiene represents a greater risk of further disease progression than a subject with periodontitis and poor oral hygiene.

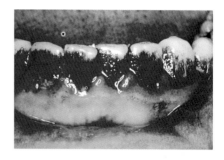

Fig 4-5 Some formal recording of hygiene levels is important medico-legally, but from a patient motivation standpoint, disclosing is essential and dichotomous chart recording of "presence/absence" is essential.

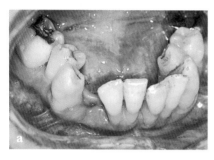
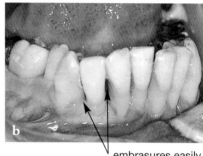

embrasures easily cleansible

Fig 4-6 An adhesive bridge designed to enable good interproximal plaque control in a periodontitis patient, currently on successful maintenance having quit a smoking habit and after full-mouth-open debridement.

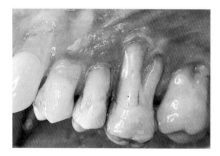
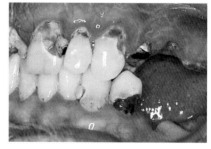

Fig 4-7 This subject has no pocketing or BOP, but excessive force during oral hygiene has resulted in attachment loss and a very large surface area to retain plaque free. The UL 6 has required root canal therapy.

Fig 4-8 This subject demonstrates extreme oral neglect, but has no periodontal bone loss or pocketing. He/she is apparently resistant to periodontitis.

- Examination of levels of plaque-retentive factors (heavily restored mouth, quality of restorations, levels of calculus).
- Presence of removable prosthesis. A well-designed bridge is less plaque retentive and more desirable than a removable partial denture (Fig 4-6).
- Levels of recession. The greater the degree of recession, the greater the surface area to clean and hence the greater risk of leaving plaque (Fig 4-7).
- Gingival tissue quality and extent of pocketing relative to levels of plaque in the mouth (Fig 4-8). Some patients appear resistant to periodontitis.

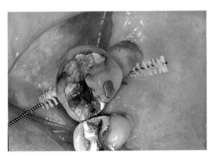

Fig 4-9 Furcation lesions require special cleaning aids to maintain plaque free.

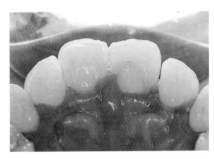

Fig 4-10 Talon cusps retain plaque close to the gingival margin.

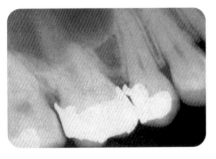

Fig 4-11 A ledged restoration with associated bone loss.

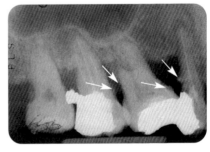

Fig 4-12 Subgingival calculus, whilst inert, can retain plaque and toxins subgingivally, causing local bone defects in susceptible patients.

Tooth-level risk assessment

Tooth-level risk assessment may or may not be carried out at the initial examination, once a BPE screen had identified a susceptible patient. In the latter situation, detailed periodontal charts and a detailed radiographic assessment and radiological report should be performed (Chapters 8 and 9). Part of this assessment would include:

- Individual tooth mobility (mobility index). Excessive mobility may compromise patient function or make a tooth susceptible to sub-luxation.
- Tooth movement or drifting. Periodontally compromised teeth may move under parafunction, a situation often seen with maxillary anterior teeth and a common presenting complaint.
- Residual tooth support (radiographically). The extent of residual radiographic bone support helps determine long-term prognosis. Chronically infected teeth with minimal bone support are best extracted to reduce the potential pathogen reservoir, which may re-infect treated and stable sites.
- Presence, location and extent of furcation lesions. Furcations (Fig 4-10) are harder to maintain and teeth should be vitality tested.
- Individual tooth anatomy (e.g. presence of "talon cusps" or bulbous crowns (Fig 4-11)).
- Anatomy of tooth embrasures and contact points (food packing, cleansability).
- Presence of ledges or deficiencies on restorations – retain plaque at or below the gingival margin (Fig 4-12).
- Individual occlusal contacts (prematurities, excessive loading, non-working-side contacts, etc.).
- Soft tissue contours.
- Subgingival calculus (Fig 4-13).

Some of the above, e.g. occlusal factors or individual contact points, may be assessed after the initial phase of therapy, where oral hygiene and scaling have

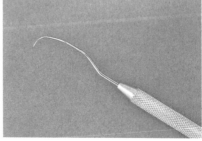

Fig 4-13 An "Old Dominican university" (ODU) explorer is useful for fine exploration of non-responder sites.

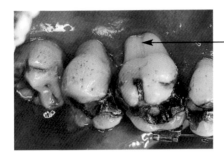

root groove

Fig 4-14 A mid-palatal root groove, exposed during surgery after repeated attempts at a non-surgical approach to therapy failed.

resolved significant areas of inflammation, but individual teeth remain resistant to this initial therapy.

Site-level risk assessment
Site-level risk assessment would include:
- Bleeding on probing. Approximately 20%–30% of BOP sites are active, whereas close to 100% of sites that repeatedly fail to BOP are inactive. However, smoking status may affect these statistics.
- Suppuration. Suppuration from a treated pocket indicates the site is unstable and either re-treatment is indicated, or an infected root canal may be present.
- Local root grooves or root concavities. Sites that fail to respond to initial therapy should be carefully explored for root grooves or cracks (Fig 4-13).
- Individual probing pocket depths. These represent historical disease rather than current activity, but the aim of therapy is to reduce pocket depths to < 4mm.
- Attachment levels.
- Other anatomical factors (e.g. enamel pearls, root grooves (Fig 4-14)).

Site-level analysis would normally follow the hygiene and scaling phase of therapy and precede root-surface debridement of those specific sites that require it. The site-characteristics at the start of maintenance are the key reference point from which to monitor site stability.

Patient-Level or Systemic Risk Factors

Patient-level or systemic risk factors can be broadly categorised as:

A. Genetic/inherited/inborn risk factors – e.g. inherited but mild defects in PMNL function can lead to significant malfunction in the presence of certain periodontal pathogens (Chapter 2), which produce toxins to disable/destroy PMNLs.

B. Environmental risk factors – e.g. drug therapies involving phenytoin (e.g. Dilantin®), used to treat epilepsy, calcium channel blockers (e.g. amlodipine), used to treat hypertension and angina, or ciclosporin, used posttransplantation to prevent organ rejection.

C. Behavioural risk factors – e.g. smoking, which is now recognised as a highly significant risk factor for periodontal disease.

D. Life-style risk factors – e.g. psychosocial stress, which is a strong risk factor for NUG (Chapter 6). Evidence is emerging that stress is also a potential risk factor for chronic periodontitis.

E. Metabolic risk factors – e.g. diabetes mellitus types I and II, which significantly enhance susceptibility to periodontitis.

F. Haematological risk factors – e.g. leucocyte adhesion deficiencies (LADs) or lazy leucocyte syndromes.

Certain risk factors may appear to be of dual classification. For example, diabetes has a strong genetic basis, but the diabetic state per se may not be the risk factor for periodontitis, rather the hyperglycaemic state, which alters PMNL function and connective tissue and lipid metabolism.

Genetic risk factors for periodontitis

There is good evidence from twin, sibling-pair and family studies that a familial pattern exists with certain forms of aggressive periodontitis. The pattern of transmission is consistent with Mendelian inheritance of a major gene or linked genes, in an autosomal dominant manner. However, the underlying risk factors remain largely obscure and are poorly understood. Furthermore, the genes responsible for such susceptibility may differ between races and continents, since PMNL defects found in one population of aggressive periodontitis patients have not been reproduced in others. Nevertheless, knowledge of a family history of aggressive periodontitis helps the practitioner to design regular recall programmes and to increase the level of detail of examinations performed at such recalls. Early diagnosis of attachment loss and active pocket formation greatly simplifies therapy.

More recently, attention has focused on single nucleotide polymorphism (SNP) analysis. SNPs are variable regions in a gene structure that essentially differ by one nucleotide only. This can result in the production of proteins of differing effectiveness. Where such a protein is a PMNL-receptor or pro-inflammatory cytokine, the effect on the inflammatory-immune response can be substantial and may play a role in determining the increased susceptibility of an individual to periodontitis (see Box 4-1). It seems logical that gene polymorphisms that are common in the population are unlikely to explain a disease like periodontitis, which is relatively uncommon (10–15% of the population). Work has therefore begun to determine the clinical effects of different combinations of the various gene polymorphisms that are currently known about. Table 4.1 summarises some genetically inherited disorders, where periodontitis is a feature, due to qualitative or quantitative defects in leucocytes.

Table 4-1 **Inherited conditions affecting the periodontal tissues**

Condition	Underlying Defect of Periodontal Relevance
Down syndrome	Defects of PMNL chemotaxis, killing and phagocytosis. Depressed T-cell antigen–induced killing.
Chronic granulomatous disease	Failure of the "respiratory burst" in phagocytes. Oxygen radicals are not produced and bacteria survive.
Insulin–dependent juvenile diabetes	Hyperglycaemic state reduces PMNL function. Monocytes are hyper-reactive and excess IL-1β, PGE$_2$, TNF-α and oxygen radicals are produced. Effects also on collagen solubility and vascularity reduce healing.
Hypophosphatasia	Low levels of the enzyme alkaline phosphatase result in poor mineralisation/formation of cementum and teeth exfoliate.
Papillon–Lefèvre syndrome	Defects of PMNL chemotaxis and phagocytosis. Gene mapped to PMNL-enzyme (Cathepsin-C) gene locus on chromosome 11.
Ehlers Danlos syndrome	Defects of collagen synthesis - Type VIII is associated with severe periodontal destruction.
Chediak–Higashi syndrome	Defects of phagocyte chemotaxis, degranulation and membrane fusion. Total loss of adult dentition.
Jobs syndrome	Excessive IgE and histamine release by mast cells and IgE immune complex formation.

Box 4-1

Examples of SNPs Investigated in Periodontitis

In 1996, Wilson and Kalmar examined a polymorphism in the PMNL-receptor that binds IgG2, the so-called FcgRIIa (Fc-gamma receptor IIa). Two allotypes exist, a high-affinity receptor (H131 – arginine coded for at position 131 on chromosome) and a low-affinity receptor (R131 – histidine coded for at position 131). They found that Black sufferers of localised early-onset (aggressive) periodontitis had an increased frequency of the low-affinity receptor, resulting in their PMNLs binding poorly to IgG2. Kornman *et al.* investigated a SNP in the IL-1 gene locus in 1997 and demonstrated that periodontitis was associated with a specific genotype (haplotype IL1-α^{-889} [allele 2] with IL1-β^{+3953} [allele 2]) that coded for excessive IL1 production. They called this the PST(+) genotype and showed that it was associated with increased susceptibility to chronic periodontitis in a small group of volunteers. A finger-prick blood test is now available for chair-side analysis. However, this polymorphism appeared predictive only for subjects who also smoked, and when applied to larger numbers of subjects, its power as a diagnostic tool reduced considerably. Similar studies in a UK population have failed to demonstrate such a relationship.

Environmental risk factors for periodontitis

Drugs such as:
- phenytoin (50%)
- calcium channel blockers (e.g. nifedipine, amlodipine, felodipine) (5%–20%)
- ciclosporin (30%)

can lead to drug-induced gingival overgrowth, false pocketing and subsequently true pocketing. It is often possible to change a patient's anti-hypertensive drug regime through their medical practitioner to a non-calcium channel blocker, which should be the first approach. One of the few indications for withdrawal of ciclosporin in transplant patients and substitution with an alternative (e.g. tacrolimus) is gingival overgrowth; again this can be achieved through consultation with the physician responsible for the transplant patient's medical control.

HIV disease
Research has demonstrated that whilst conditions such as necrotising ulcerative gingivitis (NUG), necrotising ulcerative periodontitis (NUP) and necrotising stomatitis (NS) are more common in HIV-positive patients (Chapter 6), baseline attachment levels in chronic periodontitis are no different to sero-negative controls. Additionally, attachment loss does not appear to progress at a significantly higher rate in HIV-infected over non-infected controls, provided oral hygiene is comparable.

Behavioural risk factors for periodontitis

The two most important behavioural risk factors for periodontal diseases are:
• poor oral hygiene
• smoking.

Poor oral hygiene as a risk factor
The issue of oral hygiene is the most important factor in periodontal disease. As indicated in Fig 4-2, many studies have demonstrated significant reductions in probing pocket depths, attachment gains and, of course, in gingival inflammation, with improvements in oral hygiene alone. The patient's ability to clean effectively and their motivation to do so are separate issues. However, dextrous patients who understand that their level of oral hygiene needs to be higher than that of the 90% of the population that are not at risk from periodontitis have a duty of care to themselves, which only they can fulfil on a daily basis. It is essential to motivate and monitor levels of oral hygiene by recording plaque and bleeding scores and to feed these back to the patient. The patient who repeatedly fails to achieve the levels of cleaning necessary for optimal periodontal health must accept the likelihood of disease progression and is more suited to a palliative treatment regime to maintain their dentition for as long as possible.

Smoking as a risk factor
A considerable body of evidence now supports smoking as one of the most significant risk factors for periodontal disease. The effects of tobacco smoking on the periodontium are broad and smokers:
• have more sites with deeper pockets
• have greater levels of clinical attachment loss/bone loss
• have a higher prevalence of furcation lesions
• accumulate more calculus
• demonstrate a dose response between smoking habit (pack years = num-

ber of packs per day x number of years patient has smoked) and periodontal destruction.

The link with periodontal diseases was first established in 1946 owing to an association between smoking and NUG. Ironically, nicotine and other agents within smoke cause vasoconstriction, reducing gingival bleeding and gingival redness (also owing to surface keratinistion of gingivae), and hence mask important clinical signs of periodontal inflammation.

Smokers have three to six times (depending on criteria) the level of periodontal disease of non-smokers, and 19–30-year-olds are four times more likely to suffer. Studies have shown that one cigarette per day increases attachment loss by 0.5%, ten per day by 5% and 20 per day by 10%. Ninety per cent of refractory periodontitis cases (Chapter 6) are smokers (compared with 25% of general population).

Non-surgical therapy and surgical therapy are less effective in smokers, who are two times more likely to lose teeth during periodontal maintenance. Whilst the periodontal tissues do improve with therapy, smokers experience:
- less probing pocket depth reduction
- less clinical attachment gain
- less bone height gain.

The mechanisms underlying smoking as a risk factor are complex, but may include:
- ↑ prevalence of *B. forsythus (Bf)*
- Harder to eradicate *Aa, Pg and Bf*
- ↓ levels of salivary IgA
- ↓ serum IgG_2 in smokers with early-onset disease (aggressive)
- ↓ release of lysosomal enzymes and oxygen radicals by phagocytes
- ↓ ratio of T-helper: T-suppresser cells
- ↑ release of TNFα, IL1-β, IL-6 by monocytes when stimulated by LPS
- ↓ gingival blood flow initially (may compensate/self-correct in chronic smokers)
- ↑ destruction of extra-cellular matrix proteins
- ↑ gingival keratosis and fibrosis.

Smokeless tobaccos (snuff and chewing tobacco) are associated with attachment loss adjacent to the site of chewing (mainly buccal of mandibular molars).

Cessation of smoking improves response to therapy to mid-way between non-smokers and smokers, though figures vary from one to ten years for the full benefits to be realised. The role of the dental team in smoking cessation counselling is becoming high profile, as most patients visit their dental practitioner every six months, but visit their GP relatively rarely. Two groups – females and young adults – where a smoking habit remains a major problem, in particular, regularly make use of dental services. Indeed, a two-minute, chair-side saliva test for major nicotine metabolites has been developed in our laboratories and those of collaborators. A study performed in general dental practice demonstrated significant improvements in six-week quit rates, when this was used as an adjunct to smoking cessation advice given by a general dental practitioner.

Life-style risk factors for periodontitis

The roles of psychosocial stress and to a lesser extent diet and nutrition have recently attracted attention in periodontal research.

Stress as a risk factor for periodontitis
A number of studies have investigated stress, distress and coping behaviours as risk factors for periodontal disease. Associations are difficult to make, because financial strain and depression reduce dental attendance rates and oral health awareness, hence increased levels of disease may be due to oral neglect rather than biological reasons. However, the link between NUG and stress is well established and stress does reduce immune function. Stress has also been shown to reduce saliva flow and to increase salivary viscosity, acidity and glycoprotein content, thus favouring greater plaque formation. More recently, elevated levels of noradrenaline and adrenaline, due to chronic stress, have been shown to reduce gingival blood flow. Work in our own laboratories has shown that certain periodontal pathogens can utilise these catecholamines within GCF to help them multiply, aiding survival in the hostile, iron-restrictive environment of the gingival crevice. Stress remains a potential risk factor for periodontitis.

Malnutrition as a risk factor for periodontitis
Very little research has addressed the role of the diet in periodontal disease pathogenesis. Individual vitamins (vitamin C) have been shown to affect gingival bleeding and recent work has shown improved PMNL function with citrus fruit intake, but work is needed to assess the effects of a balanced diet and complexes of antioxidants, rather than individual ones. Given the role of oxygen radicals in periodontal tissue destruction, antioxidants would seem

a good target for future research. At present, diet is only a potential risk factor for periodontitis.

Metabolic diseases/disorders as risk factors for periodontitis

This list includes:
- diabetes mellitus
- pregnancy and the oral contraceptive
- osteoporosis
- Crohn's disease
- sarcoidosis.

The effects of sex hormones during puberty and pregnancy on gingival inflammation are well recognised. Higher levels of gingivitis due to sex hormone increases during pregnancy are also recognised, but links to accelerated bone loss may be secondary to gingival inflammation, or due to behavioural changes in oral hygiene practices. Early evidence suggests a link between osteoporosis and alveolar crestal height loss, but again this may be a manifestation of a more generalised osteopenia.

Diabetes mellitus as a risk factor for periodontitis

Type I (formerly insulin-dependent) and type II (formerly non-insulin-dependent, age-onset, diet-controlled) diabetics are at increased risk for periodontitis and other oral infections, where diabetic control is poor. Specifically:
- Incidence of periodontitis post-puberty ↑ with age.
- The greater the systemic complications of diabetes the more severe the periodontitis.

The relationship with diabetes appears independent of plaque control or calculus.

Long-term diabetic control (over 30–90 days) is measured by assessing glycated haemoglobin (Hb) levels, since hyperglycaemia causes glucose irreversibly to bind to Hb. One of two types of Hb can be assessed:
- HbA1 – normal test levels <8% of Hb.
- HbA1c – normal levels 6.0–6.5% of Hb.

Type-I diabetics have:
- ↑ risk of developing periodontal disease with ↑ age.
- Disease severity ↑ with ↑ duration of diabetic condition.

- The higher the HbA1/HBA1c level the worse the bone loss, especially at interproximal sites.

Type II diabetes has largely been studied in relation to periodontal disease in a population of Pima Indians where the incidence of type II disease is high. Results show:
- Three times greater likelihood of CAL and bone loss.
- Younger Pima Indians with diabetes had five times more periodontal disease.
- Younger subjects were four times more likely to experience disease progression.
- Where glycaemic control was poor, the risk was 11-fold higher for periodontitis.

Factors that appear to contribute to the risk in diabetic patients include:
- PMNL function – impaired chemotaxis, phagocytosis and adherence have been demonstrated. The PMNL defects may be genetically inherited or may be secondary to the hyperglycaemia.
- Collagen metabolism – gingival fibroblasts from diabetic subjects synthesise less collagen and levels of PMNL collagenase are $\uparrow$.
- AGE products – in a hyperglycaemic environment protein structures undergo non-enzymatic glycation to form advanced glycation end (AGE) products. AGE products cause $\uparrow$ collagen x-linkage and thus $\downarrow$ solubility/turnover. Also, monocytes/macrophages have AGE-receptors, which when bound by AGE products stimulate release of IL-1, TNFα, PGE$_2$ and oxygen radicals.
- Wound healing – is $\downarrow$ in diabetics due to the $\downarrow$ collagen solubility and $\uparrow$ collagenase removal of newly formed collagen.

Practical points
Whilst most type I diabetics are diagnosed prior to dental attendance, type II diabetes can still present initially to the dental surgeon. The patient in Fig 4-15a presented with an atypical lateral periodontal abscess, which did not respond to simple drainage and root surface debridement. The use of urinalysis strips (Fig 4-15b) within the surgery demonstrated high urinary glucose levels and a subsequent random blood glucose test (random rather than fasting glucose as patient had eaten within the previous eight hours) demonstrated marked hyperglycaemia.

In general, the better the diabetic control the better the response to periodontal therapy. Well-controlled diabetics can be treated as any other pa-

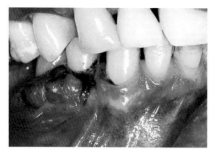

Fig 4-15 (a) Multiple lateral periodontal abscesses in an undiagnosed diabetic.

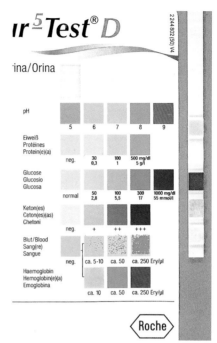

(b) Example of multi-test *urinalysis strips for in-surgery use.*

tient, but stressful procedures are probably best performed early morning, as endogenous corticosteroid levels are highest at this time. Prolonged stressful dentistry may require modification of insulin or tablet regimes to raise blood glucose levels prior to the therapy. Liaison with the patient's doctor is recommended. There is no indication for the use of antibiotics during routine periodontal therapy for diabetics; however, low dose doxycycline may inhibit PMNL collagenases and assist healing in refractory cases.

Haematological risk factors for periodontitis

A variety of haematological diseases can affect the periodontal tissues. These include:
- acute/chronic myeloid leukaemia
- myelodysplasia syndrome
- agranulocytosis
- cyclical or benign/familial neutropenia
- hypo/agammaglobulinaemia
- defects of lymphocyte formation (Di George syndrome, Wiscott-Aldrich syndrome).

69

Such conditions are rare and best referred for advice/therapy due to potential bleeding problems and those related to poor PMNL function.

Summary

Risk assessment is an important part of modern-day periodontal practice. Risk factors for acquiring periodontal disease include:
- family history
- smoking
- medical problems such as diabetes mellitus.

Risk factors for disease progression include:
- severity of existing attachment loss in relation to age
- whole mouth bleeding on probing at >25% of sites
- pockets >4mm in depth
- poorly controlled diabetes
- smoking
- plaque at >30% of sites
- local plaque-retention factors
- stress
- (possibly) poor nutrition.

It is recommended that systemic (patient-based) risk factors are documented alongside the diagnosis in patients case records.

Further Reading

Kinane DF, Chestnutt IG. Smoking and periodontal disease. Crit Rev Oral Biol Med 2000;11:356-365.

Offenbacher S. Periodontal diseases: pathogenesis. Ann Periodontol 1996;1:821-878.

Salvi GE, Lawrence HP, Offenbacher S, Beck JD. Influence of risk factors on the pathogenesis of periodontitits. Periodontology 2000. 1997;14:173-201.

Chapter 5

Natural History and Clinical Signs of Periodontal Diseases

Aim

This chapter aims to explain the changing paradigm of the natural history of periodontitis and to help the reader visualise the important clinical features of periodontal health and disease.

Outcome

The outcome of reading this chapter should be that the reader will understand how untreated periodontitis differs in its pattern of progression from treated disease, and will be able to recognise the salient features of gingival and periodontal diseases in their patients.

Natural History Studies

The natural history of a disease describes the pattern of behaviour of the disease process with time, in the absence of clinical intervention. Natural history studies are essential to our understanding of how a disease should behave and help to plan health care and improve clinical outcomes. In periodontal diseases, the ultimate treatment outcome is the retention of teeth in a state of comfort and function for life. This is the primary outcome measure of successful periodontal care, but is very difficult to measure, as teeth may be lost for many reasons and retrospective studies of tooth loss are often unable to determine with certainty the cause of the tooth loss. Secondary outcome measures are therefore often used. These would include:
- lack of tooth mobility or mobility compatible with comfortable function
- BOP at < 25% of sites
- no pocketing >4mm at any sites
- no suppuration from the gingival crevice at any sites
- plaque scores in the range of 20%–40% or less
- stable or improved CALs.

It is important to realise that decisions on ideal outcome goals must be made on an individual basis, since a target of <25% whole mouth plaque may be compatible with stability for one patient, but others may need to achieve levels <10%. Patients are likely to add to the above outcomes their own measures of success, such as:

- minimal recession
- no sensitivity
- good aesthetics
- no gingival redness
- no malodour, etc.

Harold Löe and colleagues, who examined a population of Sri Lankan tea workers who had no access to dental care, performed one of the classical natural history studies. Such population studies are important in helping identify risk factors (Chapter 4) for the disease under scrutiny and are either cross-sectional (i.e. looking for comparisons between populations at one moment in time) or longitudinal (longitudinal studies help link cause to effect and allow disease progression to be assessed). The Sri Lankan tea-worker study took place over a 15-year period and found higher disease prevalence in the tea workers than a control population in Norway. Despite the fact that the tea workers had large amounts of plaque and calculus the progression rate for disease was:

8% in a rapid-progression group (high-risk group)

81% progressed at a moderate rate (medium-risk group)

11% showed no progression and were apparently disease resistant.

These figures are now regarded as being on the high side, owing to the methods used to define disease presence and progression, but, nevertheless, worldwide studies support figures of between 5% and 15% of the population being at risk from severe destruction in adult life. The statistics for early-onset (aggressive) diseases are closer to 1% of Caucasian subjects below the age of 25 years being at risk of significant destruction and up to 3% of Asian and Afro-Caribbean subjects. However, more recent studies by Clerehugh and colleagues have identified progression of attachment loss, albeit slow, in 77% of 167 adolescents aged 14–19 years at some point over a five-year observation period. The attachment loss was related to high levels of plaque and calculus. Nevertheless, whilst a minority of the population appears to be at risk of total tooth loss from periodontitis, a significant number may experience some tooth loss owing to disease that starts at a younger age than previously thought. Periodontitis is believed to account for 35% of all tooth loss.

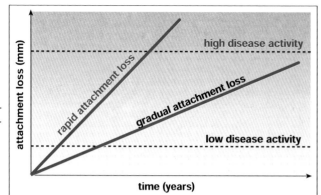

Fig 5-1 The "linear model" for periodontal disease progression assumes constant disease activity at different rates for different individuals.

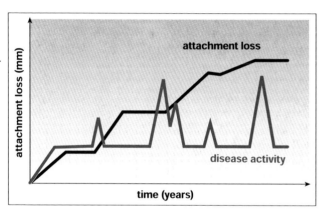

Fig 5-2 The "random burst or multiple asynchronous burst" model of Socransky and colleagues assumes periods of activity and remission. The latter vary in number and size, both between and within individuals.

Linear Disease Progression Versus the Burst Theory

Until the early 1980s, periodontal disease progression was thought to follow a linear pattern with time (Fig 5-1). High-risk individuals would lose attachment at a rapid rate owing to a higher level of disease activity than lower-risk individuals. However, a series of studies performed between 1982 and 1984 in Boston changed the traditional paradigm and the *random burst and multiple asynchronous burst* hypotheses were born (Fig 5-2). Goodson and colleagues examined 22 subjects by manual probing of six sites per tooth, every two months for a year. They estimated the errors involved in their probing and set thresholds above this error (around 2.5mm) to signify a real change in attachment level. They determined that the disease process appeared to follow a more random pattern than previously thought where periods of active disease were interspersed with periods of inactivity and repair. The number and magnitude of episodes differed both between and within individual subjects, and sometimes occurred in multiple asynchronous bursts. Some claimed that the high thresholds used in these studies favoured the finding of a more unpredictable pattern of attachment loss. In 1991, a study by a group in Alabama utilised an electronic probe which measured to a degree of accuracy of 0.1mm (i.e. smaller increments) and found linear disease progression in 76% of their 30 subjects. However, they used a threshold arguably too low (active disease was found at 29% of sites – a high figure) and their analysis method favoured a linear model. The outcome of these studies was that there appeared to be a subgroup of the periodontitis-prone population in whom disease progression was discontinuous and unpredictable (about 25%).

Several studies during the 1990s added to the body of knowledge by assessing the pattern of disease progression using larger subject numbers and different study designs. Taken together, the studies broadly fall into two groups:
• Studies of un-treated disease – which demonstrate a burst type pattern of progress.
• Studies of treated disease during maintenance – which show a more linear pattern of disease progression.

The above outcome seems logical, given that untreated disease has many contributing local and behavioural risk factors, and one would thus expect an unpredictable pattern of progression. Once risk factors are corrected and causative agents (plaque) controlled, it may be expected that any disease that progresses is likely to follow a more predictable pattern.

Disease Markers

The random burst theory stimulated a lot of research work aimed at identifying markers of *disease activity*, which were superior to existing clinical measures. Many such markers measured in GCF achieved 80% sensitivity for diagnosis (true positive diagnoses) and 80% specificity (true negative diagnoses), with positive and negative predictive values for the development of active disease >75%. Whilst these were far superior to individual clinical measures, they were too cumbersome for dental practice, and at present they look unlikely to become accepted as standard practice. This chapter will therefore focus on clinical markers of disease. It is important to remember that the experienced clinician takes a large number of such measures into account before deciding on whether a patient or site requires active therapy. No study has attempted to quantify the effectiveness of this approach in terms of diagnostic accuracy, because there are simply too many variables to account for, and volunteer numbers would need to be enormous in such studies.

Clinical Signs of Pristine Periodontal Health

Fig 1-2 is a picture of classical pristine periodontal health. Its features are:

1. Pink gingivae (there are individual differences; some may show racial pigmentation).
2. Firm gingivae (no swelling).
3. Uniform colour (no patches of marked redness).
4. Presence of stippling (referred to as "orange peel effect").
5. A knife-edged gingival margin.
6. Intact gingival margin (no ulceration).
7. A flat and triangular interdental papilla (normally filling inderdental space).
8. A probing depth <3mm, when 20-25g weight is applied to the probe.
9. Complete absence of any bleeding to probe.
10. Complete absence of any suppuration (pus).
11. A gingival margin situated just above the CEJ.
12. Complete absence of furcation exposure.
13. No recession.

It is important to remember, however, that clinical gingival health may not be classical (Fig 1-9). For example, teeth spaced apart may have a flattened interdental papilla. In addition, attachment loss may occur owing to toothbrush trauma and recession may be consistent with health, albeit not classical health. Following periodontal therapy, there may be reduced support, exposed furcations, residual drifting and mobility, but the disease may no longer be active and hence the tissues are clinically healthy at that time (Fig 5-3). Indeed, age-related changes such as recession and changes in soft-tis-

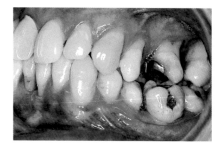

Fig 5-3 Clinical health in a patient post-therapy who had been stable for seven years and required no more than occasional calculus removal.

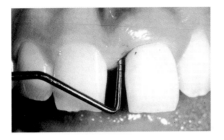

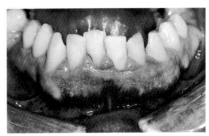

Fig 5-4 Deep pocketing present, with very subtle signs of inflammation to the untrained eye. This would be easily missed unless routine periodontal probing is performed.

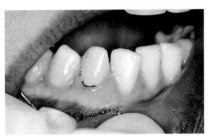

Fig 5-5 Early signs of gingival inflammation, mild rolling of marginal tissues and loss of stippling.

Fig 5-6 Chronic gingivitis of several months' duration, with fibrosis and oedema present.

sue consistency result in healthy periodontal tissues in the elderly failing to satisfy the conditions of classical or "pristine" health.

Clinical Signs of Gingivitis

It is largely accepted that gingivitis precedes periodontitis, even though gingivitis does not always lead to periodontitis and periodontal pocketing can develop in the absence of obvious inflammation (Fig 5-4). However, the classical features of inflamed gingival tissues are:

1. Redness (starting at the papilla and progressing along the margin).
2. Loss of stippling.
3. Swelling (oedema) – with which the tissues become softer and "pit" on pressing.
4. Rolling of the gingival margin and loss of the triangular shape of the interdental papilla.
5. Bleeding on gentle probing.

Fig 5-5 shows early gingivitis, whereas Fig 5-6 demonstrates a more chronic and established inflammatory state, where the body's attempts at healing

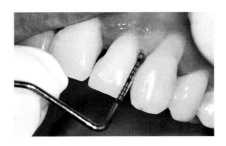

Fig 5-7 Classical periodontitis measured using University of North Carolina 15mm (UNC-15) probe.

have led to fibrosis. False pocketing may arise with gingivitis, where the probing pocket depth exceeds 3mm, but the JE remains at the CEJ (Fig 1-3).

Clinical Signs of Periodontitis

Accepting that sites of periodontal disease may not necessarily demonstrate all the signs of gingivitis, classical features of periodontitis (Fig 5-7) are:
– some or all of the signs of gingivitis (see above)
– true pocketing on probing, i.e. probing pocket depths ≥4mm, where the pocket base is apical to the CEJ (i.e. attachment loss has occurred)
– recession
– suppuration
– mobility above physiological levels (>0.2mm)
– drifting of teeth
– exposure of furcations
– radiographic evidence of bone loss.

Historical Verses Active Disease

The principal limitation of clinical measures of periodontal disease is that they measure disease experience rather than current disease activity. For example, radiographic bone loss and clinical attachment loss provide measures of the cumulative effects of periodontal damage, up to a point within the recent past. The importance of determining whether a site is active or inactive is that instrumentation of inactive sites can lead to attachment loss due to the trauma of instrumentation. It is important therefore to determine the need for therapy on a site-by-site basis, taking into account all available information for that site.

Scenario 1
A 6mm pocket that does not bleed when probed nor exhibit pus discharge,

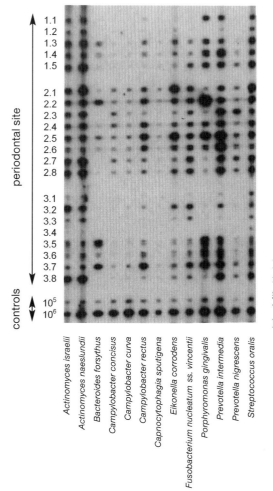

Fig 5-8 Checkerboard immunoblot showing which organisms were detected at individual sites within the same patient.

and within which subgingival deposits cannot be detected, should not be instrumented, but simply reviewed after four to six months. If the 6mm pocket remains stable, subgingival prophylaxis may be the only therapy indicated.

Scenario 2
A 6mm pocket presenting as for scenario 1, but with detectable subgingival calculus, should be scaled subgingivally and reviewed after three to four months.

Scenario 3

A 6mm pocket presenting as in scenario 1, but with bleeding on probing, should be root debrided and reviewed three to four months later.

In all cases, care must be taken to ensure that no subgingival local risk factors exist.

Concept of Site-Specificity

The final concept to consider in relation to clinical signs of health/disease and patterns of disease progression is that of site-specificity. This simply means that the micro-flora, the anatomy, the local immune response, etc. at one site around one tooth, may be totally different from an adjacent site of the same tooth. This is best illustrated with a checkerboard immunoblot (Fig 5-8). The immunoblot is a research tool which uses DNA probes to as many species as necessary and cross-binds the probes to the complementary bacterial DNA in a plaque sample. In Fig 5-8, each vertical column represents a particular organism and each horizontal row represents a plaque sample from a single site. Where a black spot appears, the organism is present at that site. The profile for the site sampled on tooth 1.1 is very different from that for 1.3, from the same tooth in the same patient. The relevance of this is that periodontal therapy must be based upon site-specific data derived from detailed charts and not on "whole mouth" appearances (see Chapter 8).

Further Reading

Clerehugh V, Worthington HV, Lennon MA, Chandler R. Site progression of loss of attachment over 5 years in 14- to 19-year-old adolescents. J Clin Periodontol 1995;22:15-21.

Goodson JM, Tanner AC, Haffajee AD, Sornberger GC, Socransky SS. Patterns of progression and regression of advanced destructive periodontal disease. J Clin Periodontol 1982;9:472-481.

Löe H, Anerud A, Boyson H, Smith M. The natural history of periodontal disease in man. The rate of periodontal destruction before 40 years of age. J Periodontol 1978;49:607-620.

Socransky SS, Haffajee AD, Goodson JM, Lindhe J. New concepts of destructive periodontal disease. J Clin Periodontol 1984;11:21-32.

Chapter 6

Classification of Periodontal Diseases

Aim

This chapter aims to explain the necessity for classification systems and how such systems have evolved in periodontology to the present day. The faults with existing systems will be highlighted and a simplified classification proposed for general dental practice.

Outcome

The outcome of reading this chapter should be that the practitioner understands the chronological relationship between old and current diagnostic terms in periodontology, and is able to introduce a logical system of classification into their own clinical practice.

Why Do We Need Classification Systems?

This chapter is the simplest in the book in terms of concepts, but proved the hardest to write, owing to the broad controversy that surrounds classification systems for periodontal diseases.

Traditionally, classification systems were simple. Owing to a paucity of knowledge and evidence from research, little was known about these diseases and thus simple terms were applied, by necessity. During the 1970s, 1980s and early 1990s, research into periodontal diseases exploded and our knowledge base broadened dramatically. The classification categories of the 1970s, 1980s and early 1990s therefore expanded to encompass new diseases for which there was putative evidence, based largely on case reports. However, there are important differences between having knowledge and having understanding. As a consequence (as with most things in the modern world), the wheel has turned almost full circle and the 1999 International Workshop on Periodontal Disease Classification has re-reduced the number of common disease categories – reflecting our lack of genuine understanding of these complex diseases and what differentiates them – and increased the number of less-common disease categories.

Classification systems are essential, largely because without them it is not possible to arrive at an informed diagnosis. Without a robust diagnosis, appropriate therapy cannot be implemented. Classification systems also:

- Direct research aimed at learning more about the diseases concerned.
- Help determine the evidence base for better-targeted therapy.
- Guide practitioners towards the best method for treating a disease.
- Enable the international community to communicate in a common language.
- Guide public health planning and targeting of therapy.
- Help practitioners plan treatment protocols to maximise benefit to all their patients.

Basic Terms that Appear in Such Systems

When designing classification systems, a series of traditional terms is often used as the basis for sub-categorisation.

Acute

The term "acute" is one of the most frequently used in medical disease classification. "Acute" is a term that describes a short-lived, intense, brisk experience that is often a distressing one and is assumed to require immediate action. Recent classifications have thus removed it from the titles of diseases like AUG, which became ANUG, but has now been replaced by the term NUG. The situation is similar for the acute lateral periodontal abscess, now called a "lateral periodontal abscess". Acute diseases may often be curable, e.g. acute lymphoblastic/cytic leukaemia in children. Eliminating the infective agent can cure the majority of acute infections.

Chronic

If a disease is not acute, then by default it is a chronic process. "Chronic" diseases have a longer "time course" and are generally not immediately life-threatening. However, the evidence base for the "time course" that designates a disease acute or chronic varies from one human system to the next, and in the periodontium there is no consensus on what a short or long time course may be. Chronic diseases are generally incurable, and management involves the control of symptoms, or the prevention of more serious complications. For example, diabetes mellitus and HIV disease are managed to prevent systemic complications and prolong life-expectancy to as close to normal as possible. Rheumatoid arthritis and Crohn's disease are managed symptomatically. Periodontal diseases are largely chronic and cannot currently be cured, but they can be controlled.

Aggressive
"Aggressive" is a term that describes a rapid progression over a short period of time (months or a few years). Previously the term "rapidly progressing" was used in this manner.

Juvenile
"Juvenile" is a term used to describe a disease whose onset occurred during juvenile years.

Localised
"Localised" is a term used to designate a disease involving a small number of teeth (see below).

Generalised
"Generalised" is the term used to describe diseases involving the majority of teeth present in the mouth.

Historical Perspective pre-1999

Many different terms have been used for periodontal diseases over the years. In Sir Wilfred Fish's 1952 text, *Parodontal Disease: A Manual of Treatment and Atlas of Pathology* (2nd edn.), the diseases were classified as:

Degenerative/abnormalities of growth - these included senile alveolar resorption (osteoporotic changes), odontoclasia (root apex resorption) and hypercementosis.

Inflammations – these included traumatic inflammations, acute ulcerative stomatitis (now called NUG), sub-acute marginal gingivitis, chronic marginal gingivitis (which included drug-induced overgrowths), pyorrhoea simplex (mild periodontitis) and pyorrhoea profunda (advanced periodontitis).

Neoplasia – which included odontoclastoma, cementoma and fibrous epulis.

It can be seen from the current international system (Tables 6-1 and 6-2), how little some things have changed in fifty years!

Table 6-1 illustrates the changes in classification systems over the years. The evolutionary inter-relationships of the aggressive periodontal diseases are illustrated in Fig 6-1. Such terminology has led to a great deal of confusion and when the American Academy of Periodontology and a European Workshop produced differing systems again in the 1990s, it was time for world-wide agreement. The "International Workshop for Classification of Periodontal Diseases and Conditions" was therefore established and reported in Decem-

Table 6-1 **Classification systems through the years**

Year	Responsible Body	The System
1977	American Academy of Periodontology	juvenile periodontitis chronic marginal periodontitis
1986	American Academy of Periodontology	juvenile periodontitis (pre-pubertal) (localised) (generalised) adult periodontitis necrotising ulcerative peri- odontitis refractory periodontitis
1989	J Lindhe (ed.) *Textbook of Clinical Periodontology*, 2nd ed. Munksgard: Copenhagen, 1989.	periodontitis levis periodontitis gravis
1989	American Academy of Periodontology	early-onset periodontitis adult periodontitis periodontitis associated with systemic disease necrotising ulcerative peri- odontitis refractory periodontitis
1993	European Workshop on Periodontology	early-onset periodontitis adult periodontitis necrotising ulcerative peri- odontitis
1999	World Workshop	see Tables 6-2 and 6-3

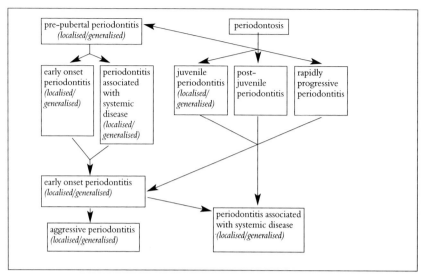

Fig 6-1 The inter-relationship between various terms used to describe aggressive forms of periodontitis over the years.

ber 1999, their current view based on the best evidence available to date. This is illustrated in Tables 6-2 and 6-3, but is unhelpfully complex, being driven, in part, by the needs of health insurance companies in the USA and parts of Europe to have designated terms against which fees can be arranged.

International Workshop for Classification of Periodontal Diseases and Conditions

The 1999 classification is still controversial, but is becoming accepted as a useful reference system, albeit too cumbersome for day-to-day general dental practice. It aimed to address some of the limitations of the 1989 system, which included:

- No category for gingival diseases/conditions.
- The term "adult periodontitis", implying that chronic periodontal attachment loss only affected adults, although there is good evidence that chronic attachment loss can affect adolescents (Chapter 5).
- Early-onset periodontitis – a term applied to disease affecting individuals <35yrs of age, even though aggressive disease can affect slightly older individuals also.

Table 6-2 **International workshop 1999 – gingival diseases**

A. Dental plaque-induced gingival diseases

    1. Gingivitis associated with dental plaque only
      a. without other local contributing factors
      b. with local contributing factors (G.1 Table 6-3)

    2. Gingival diseases modified by systemic factors
      a. associated with the endocrine system
        1) puberty-associated gingivitis
        2) menstrual cycle-associated gingivitis
        3) pregnancy-associated
          a) gingivitis
          b) pyogenic granuloma
        4) diabetes mellitus-associated gingivitis
      b. associated with blood dyscrasias
        1) leukemia-associated gingivitis
        2) other

    3. Gingival diseases modified by medications
      a. drug-influenced gingival diseases
        1) drug-influenced gingival enlargements
        2) drug-influenced gingivitis
          a) oral contraceptive-associated gingivitis
          b) other

    4. Gingival diseases modified by malnutrition
      a. ascorbic acid-deficiency gingivitis
      b. other

B. Non-plaque-induced gingival lesions

    1. Gingival diseases of specific bacterial origin
      a. Neisseria gonorrhea-associated lesions
      b. Treponema pallidum-associated lesions
      c. streptococcal species-associated lesions
      d. other

    2. Gingival diseases of viral origin
      a. herpes virus infections
        1) primary herpetic gingivostomatitis
        2) recurrent oral herpes
        3) varicella-zoster infections
      b. other

3. *Gingival diseases of fungal origin*
   a. Candida-species infections
      1) generalized gingival candidosis
      2) linear gingival erythema
      3) histoplasmosis
      4) other

4. *Gingival lesions of genetic origin*
   a. hereditary gingival fibromatosis
   b. other

5. *Gingival manifestations of systemic conditions*
   a. mucocutaneous disorders
      1) lichen planus
      2) pemphigoid
      3) pemphigus vulgaris
      4) erythema multiforme
      5) lupus erythematosus
      6) drug-induced
      7) other
   b. allergic reactions
      1) dental restorative materials
         i) mercury
         ii) nickel
         iii) acrylic
         iv) other
      2) reactions attributable to
         i) toothpastes/dentifrices
         ii) mouthrinses/mouthwashes
         iii) chewing gum additives
         iv) foods and additives
      3) other

6. *Traumatic lesions (factitious, iatrogenic, accidental)*
   a. chemical injury
   b. physical injury
   c. thermal injury

7. *Foreign body reactions*

8. *Not otherwise specified (NOS)*

Table 6-3 **International workshop 1999 – periodontal diseases**

C. Chronic periodontitis
1. *Localised*
2. *Generalised*

D. Aggressive periodontitis
1. *Localised*
2. *Generalised*

E. Periodontitis as a manifestation of systemic diseases
1. *Associated with haematological disorders*
   a. Acquired neutropenia
   b. Leukemias
   c. Other

2. *Associated with genetic disorders*
   a. Familial and cyclic neutropenia
   b. Down syndrome
   c. Leucocyte adhesion deficiency syndromes
   d. Papillon-Lefèvre syndrome
   e. Chediak-Higashi syndrome
   f. Histiocytosis syndromes
   g. Glycogen storage disease
   h. Infantile genetic agranulocytosis
   i. Cohen syndrome
   j. Ehlers-Danlos syndrome (Types IV and VIII)
   k. Hypophosphatasia
   l. Other

3. *Not otherwise specified (NOS)*

D. Necrotising periodontal diseases
1. *Necrotising ulcerative gingivitis (NUG)*
2. *Necrotising ulcerative periodontitis (NUP)*

E. Abscesses of the periodontium
1. *Gingival abscess*
2. *Periodontal abscess*
3. *Pericoronal abscess*

F. Periodontitis associated with endodontic lesions
1. *Combined periodontic-endodontic lesions*

G. Developmental or acquired deformities and conditions

1. Localised tooth-related factors that modify or predispose to plaque-induced gingival diseases/periodontitis
  a. Tooth anatomic factors
  b. Dental restorations/appliances
  c. Root fractures
  d. Cervical root resorption and cemental tears

2. Mucogingival deformities and conditions around teeth
  a. Gingival/soft tissue recession
    1) facial or lingual surfaces
    2) interproximal (papillary)
  b. Lack of keratinized gingiva
  c. Decreased vestibular depth
  d. Aberrant frenum/muscle position
  e. Gingival excess
    1) pseudopocket
    2) inconsistent gingival margin
    3) excessive gingival display
    4) gingival enlargement
  f. Abnormal colour

3. Mucogingival deformities and conditions on edentulous ridges
  a. Vertical and/or horizontal ridge deficiency
  b. Lack of gingiva/keratinised tissue
  c. Gingival/soft tissue enlargement
  d. Aberrant frenum/muscle position
  e. Decreased vestibular depth
  f. Abnormal colour

4. Occlusal trauma
  a. Primary occlusal trauma
  b. Secondary occlusal trauma

- Periodontitis associated with systemic disease –poorly defined with many of the conditions in fact periodontal manifestations of systemic diseases.

The 1999 system therefore addressed the issues above by making the following changes to previous systems:
- A category for gingival diseases was introduced.
- The term "adult" was replaced by "chronic".
- Refractory periodontitis was removed as a separate entity, since it was felt that all forms of periodontitis may rebound as recurrent disease, but that did not necessarily mean that a group of individuals existed with common biological risk factors that made them resistant to therapy.
- The term "aggressive" was introduced to replace the term "early-onset".
- Systemic diseases that can affect the periodontal tissues were more comprehensively defined.
- The term "necrotising periodontal diseases" was adopted to cover NUG and NUP, since it was unclear whether these two were separate disease entities.
- Periodontal abscess and periodontal-endodontic lesions were added.
- A category for "developmental" or "acquired" conditions was also added.

Specific Issues with the 1999 System

Replacement of "adult" with "chronic"
This move seems logical for reasons previously stated. The term "chronic" refers to the rate of progression of *untreated* disease with time and does not imply that the disease is untreatable. Treatment is aimed at stabilisation and regeneration, rather than curing the disease. It is important that patients realise that periodontal diseases cannot be cured, only controlled, and their role in that process is crucial on a day-to-day basis. The rate of progression in each individual depends upon local and systemic risk factors. External risk factors like smoking can be controlled by many patients when educated. In general terms:

> Localised disease affects <30% of sites
> Generalised disease affects >30% of sites
> Mild disease involves 1–2mm CAL
> Moderate disease involves 3–4 mm CAL
> Severe disease involves >5mm CAL.

Recurrent disease v. refractory
Refractory disease was traditionally regarded as recurrent disease in individuals who had good home care and had been treated adequately. The term

"recurrent disease" in the 1999 system can be applied to any disease category and the likelihood of it occurring is affected by factors such as:
- extent of disease
- furcation exposure
- tooth type and position
- occlusal trauma
- microflora
- host response
- smoking, etc.

The term "recurrent" implies, correctly, that anyone who has had periodontal disease can redevelop the disease if plaque control is not maintained.

Aggressive periodontitis
This term implies CAL over a short period of time irrespective of age, but in patients who are systemically healthy. In practical terms, the majority of such individuals are young when the disease first manifests and underlying biological susceptibility is present. Key characteristics include:
- patients are systemically healthy
- familial aggregation
- rapid rate of attachment and bone loss
- tissue destruction is inconsistent with levels of plaque
- *Aa* is elevated in proportion and *Pg* may be in some cases
- there may be abnormally suppressed phagocyte function
- there may be abnormally raised phagocyte function
- the condition may "burn out".

Features specific to *localised* aggressive periodontitis (Fig 6-5) are:
- circumpubertal onset
- robust serum antibody response to bacteria involved (but response may be ineffective)
- localised to 1st molar and incisor teeth, with interproximal attachment loss at 2 or more teeth and not involving more than 2 non-1st molar or incisor teeth.

Features specific to *generalised* aggressive periodontitis (Fig 6-6) are:
- usually affects patients <30yrs of age (may be older)
- poor serum antibody response to infecting organisms
- generalised interproximal attachment loss affecting at least 3 permanent teeth that are not 1st molars or incisors.

The reason it is important to specify the term interproximal attachment loss

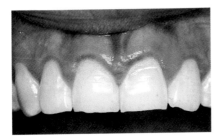

Fig 6-2 A gingival ephylis (freckle).

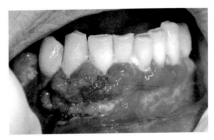

Fig 6-3 A gingival squamous cell carcinoma (SCC) arising within an area of desquamative gingivitis (presumptive diagnosis of erosive lichen planus).

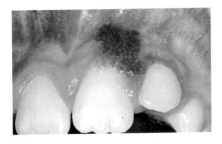

Fig 6-4 A localised viral wart caused by molluscum contageosum.

is to differentiate it from one of the most common non-plaque related causes of attachment loss, that of traumatic toothbrushing, which affects facial surfaces (mostly buccal).

Critique of the 1999 International Workshop System

The 1999 system (Table 6-3) has some plus points, but a number of negatives having succeeded largely in moving disease categories into different boxes:

- The developmental or acquired conditions/deformities are not strictly periodontal conditions, they are modifying factors that can impact on all forms of periodontitis.
- The term "aggressive" is welcomed owing to the obvious difficulties associated with a 35-years-of-age cut-off (e.g. if the patient is 36 years of age at first presentation, with severe disease, is it chronic or aggressive?). However, the loss of the association with a younger age within the title is a retrograde step, since patients in their 40s and above rarely, if ever, present with new aggressive attachment loss, unless there are recognised local or systemic risk factors associated
- The loss of the term "refractory" is regrettable. Whilst the logic behind this is clear, it is also clear that a small but specific group of individuals ex-

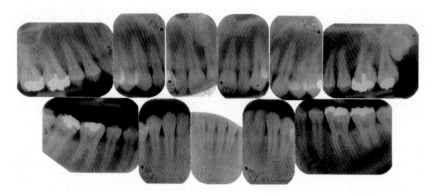

Fig 6-5 Full mouth peri-apical radiographs of localised aggressive periodontitis.

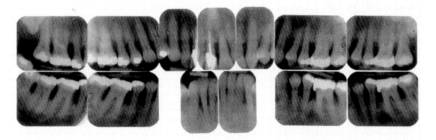

Fig 6-6 Full mouth peri-apical radiographs of generalised aggressive periodontitis.

ist who, following a high standard of therapy and with high levels of plaque control consistent with successful therapy for the majority, continue to suffer periodontal breakdown at regular intervals. There is also evidence for common underlying risk factors like smoking and specific immune defects in these patients.

- The term "necrotising periodontal diseases" is again understood, but NUG is a condition limited to the gingiva and by definition *not* involving the periodontal attachment apparatus. These terms should remain separate since the JE has not migrated apically in NUG, whilst acknowledgement should be given that NUG may or may not progress to NUP.
- The term "necrotising stomatitis" does not appear in the necrotising periodontal diseases list. However, if the criteria applied to this group are to be consistent, it should be added to this category.

- There are many conditions to affect the gingiva that are not listed, e.g. the gingival ephylis (freckle (Fig 6-2)), gingival squamous cell carcinoma (Fig 6-3), viral warts (Fig 6-4), etc. If the system aims to be comprehensive, it should be so.
- Some of the so-called "modifying factors" for plaque-related disease are not modifying factors (e.g. vitamin C deficiency and drug-induced may be plaque independent).
- Periodontitis as a manifestation of systemic diseases is strictly a misnomer. The correct term should be "periodontal manifestations of systemic diseases". Diabetes mellitus does not appear in this section, because it can affect the progression of any form of periodontitis, but if this is the case, it should appear under section G (Developmental or acquired deformities and conditions) as should smoking as "modifying factors".
- The main problem with the new classification is the loss of the term "localised juvenile periodontitis" (LJP). LJP is phenotypically the best defined of all forms of periodontitis, with clear clinical descriptors. The loss of the term from the classification system is, in the author's opinion, regrettable.

A Practical Classification for General Dental Practice

When attempting to form a diagnosis, the practitioner generally tries to determine the following questions:
- the history of the condition
- family history
- presence of subject-based risk factors (e.g. smoking)
- health or disease
- gingivitis or periodontitis
- presence, distribution and location of attachment loss
- presence, distribution and location of true pocketing
- age of patient at presentation
- apparent rate of progression
- presence, distribution and location of site-based risk factors
- radiographic evidence, pattern, amount and character of bone loss
- presence of suppuration or bleeding
- plaque levels
- degree of mobility or drifting of teeth
- occlusal factors
- is the disease *active* or in remission? (Chapter 5).

A simplified and practical classification system is outlined in Table 6-4.

Table 6-4 **Simplified classification – based on world workshop, 1999**

1. Plaque-induced gingival diseases
        a. localised –
               I. gingival abscess
               II. fibrous epulis
               III. vascular epulis
               IV. giant cell epulis
                    peripheral
                    central
        b. generalised –
               I. no modifying factors
               II. modified by sex hormones
               III. modified by medications
               IV. modified by malnutrition

2. Non plaque-induced gingival diseases
        a. specific bacterial (e.g. NUG, gonorrhoea)
        b. specific viral (e.g. 1° herpes, hand, foot and mouth)
        c. specific fungal (e.g. LGE)
        d. hereditory lesions (e.g. HGF)
        e. manifestations of systemic disease
               I. mucocutaneous disease (e.g. lichen planus/pemphigoid)
               II. allergy (e.g. toothpaste)
               III. haematological disease (e.g. leukaemia)
               IV. granulomatous disease (e.g. Crohn's, sarcoidosis)
               V. immunological disease
               VI. other
        f. tumours (e.g. SCC, KS)
        g. trauma
               I. thermal
               II. chemical
               III. physical
        h. not otherwise specified

3. Plaque-induced periodontal diseases:
        a. prepubertal periodontitis –
               I. localised
               II. generalised
        b. aggressive periodontitis –
               I. localised (LJP: see text)
               II. generalised (see text)
               III. recurrent

      c. chronic periodontitis –
          I. localised (<30% sites)
          II. generalised (>30% sites)
          III. recurrent
      d. refractory periodontitis

4. Systemic diseases affecting periodontal tissues:
      a. haematological
      b. genetic diseases
          I. neutropenia
          II. Down syndrome
          III. LAD/LLS
          IV. Chediak-Higashi syndrome
          V. hypophosphatasia
          VI. histeocytosis-X
          VII. Ehlers Danlos syndrome
          VIII. Papillon-Lefèvre syndrome
      c. not otherwise specified

5. Necrotising periodontitis:
          I. localised to periodontium
          II. necrotising stomatitis

6. Lateral periodontal abscess

7. Periodontal-endodontic lesions

Modifying factors
      These are listed in Table 6-3 under "G"

NUG = necrotising ulcerative gingivitis
LGE = linear gingival erythema
HGF = hereditary gingivo-fibromatosis
SCC = squamous cell carcinoma
KS   = Kaposi's sarcoma
LAD = leucocyte adhesion defect
LLS   = lazy leucocyte syndrome

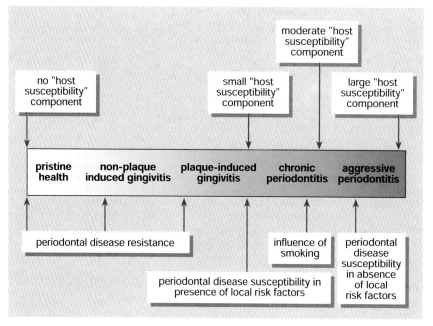

Fig 6-7 The "spectrum" of periodontal diseases, with proposed markers indicating where various factors may exert an influence.

The Ideal Classification System

Ideally, diseases should be classified according to their aetiology or pathology. For example, TB is the name given to a mono-infection with *mycobacterium tuberculosis*, HIV disease is caused by the *human immunodeficiency virus*, and myocardial infarction is what it says and is not diagnosed as "crushing chest pain". The problem with periodontal diseases is that they are polymicrobial and poly-immune/inflammatory and the exact contribution of each factor varies from one individual to the next. What is clear is that there are three categories of patient:

Category I   – Some individuals (8% ONS 1998 UK Adult Dental Health Survey) are systemically susceptible to the disease.
Category II – Some individuals can develop the disease due to local factors.
Category III – Some individuals are resistant to the disease.

It would be attractive to be able to rename localised aggressive periodontitis as localised Aa–associated periodontitis, but Aa is not always isolated from diseased sites and is often present when the clinical disease is not (see Chapter 2). For this reason, at present, periodontal diseases should be regarded as a spectrum of disease, the outcome of which is attachment loss (Fig 6-7). This model essentially relates risk to periodontal diseases in otherwise healthy individuals, i.e. pre–pubertal periodontitis and periodontal manifestations of systemic diseases/syndromes fall outside the model, as they have a clearly defined genetic basis.

Further Reading

1999 International Workshop for a Classification of Periodontal Diseases and Conditions. Annals Periodontol 1999:4;1-112.

Morris AJ, Steele J, White DA. The oral cleanliness and periodontal health of UK adults in 1998. British Dent J. 2001;191:186-192.

Chapter 7
The Initial Consultation – Screening Examination

Aim

This chapter aims to provide the practitioner with a simple algorithm for assessing and screening all patients for periodontal diseases.

Outcome

At the end of this chapter the reader should understand the importance of an accurate and comprehensive history to making a periodontal diagnosis. They should be able to screen all patients rapidly to identify those at risk of periodontal disease in the future, but should also appreciate the limitations of the screening systems recommended.

The History

When a patient first attends for consultation it is important that a thorough history and examination take place and that at subsequent visits these are competently updated. Certain historical information is essential if the clinician is to reach a correct diagnosis and develop an appropriate treatment plan. It can be subdivided as follows.

The History of the Complaint

Information gleaned from a complaint history is often extremely useful. The main points to cover are:
1. The length of time the patient has been aware of the problem.
2. Determination of whether the problem is purely localized or whether there is systemic involvement.
3. A detailed description of the symptoms, including nature, frequency, severity, duration, etc.
4. Whether the nature of the symptoms has changed with time, e.g. changes in number, frequency or severity.
5. Whether anything exacerbates or relieves the symptoms.
6. Whether the patient has received treatment for the condition and, if so, when and from whom and whether this therapy was efficacious.
7. Whether there is a family history of the problem.

The Medical History

The key questions to be asked are given in detail elsewhere and need not be repeated here. There are, however, three main reasons for collecting this information:

1. It may, in whole or in part, explain why a particular condition is seen and may account for the severity of reported/observed symptoms/signs.
2. It should alert the clinician to the existence of systemic factors for which special precautions will be required to safeguard the patient during treatment, e.g. antibiotic prophylaxis.
3. It should alert the clinician to any disease processes suffered by a patient which may present a risk both to staff in the clinical setting and to subsequent patients, e.g. Hepatitis B carrier or patient with CJD.

The Social History

Details of what should be covered are available elsewhere. A social history should include a full history of habits such as smoking and alcohol consumption. It is a concern that increased numbers of young women in particular are smoking. It is important to consider tobacco smoking carefully because:

1. Tobacco smoking causes many potentially damaging changes in the body:
   - During smoking, nicotine is rapidly absorbed into the blood stream where 30% remains in free form. It is highly lipid–soluble and thus gains easy passage across cell membranes, where it appears particularly to affect neural tissue including the brain. This may help account for the psychological dependence effects.
   - Nicotine increases heart rate, cardiac output and blood pressure. It also acts directly upon blood vessels inducing vasoconstriction.
2. Tobacco smoking also causes potentially damaging oral changes:
   - Prolonged thermal and chemical irritation of oral mucosa from smoke may result in changes in the oral mucosa ranging from relatively benign conditions such as "smoker's keratosis" and "nicotinus stomatitis" and more potentially sinister conditions such as leukoplakia through to frank carcinoma. The principal carcinogens within tobacco smoke include polycyclic aromatic hydrocarbons and N–nitroso compounds.
   - Tobacco smoke is selectively bactericidal and causes changes in the oral microflora, resulting in a predisposition to candidosis.
   - Extrinsic staining of the teeth and soft tissues occurs due to deposition of tar products. Staining of the teeth encourages plaque accumulation due to the rough surface of the stain, which may, in "risk patients", result in increased periodontal disease experience.

- Smoking is heavily implicated in the aetiology of NUG.
- Smokers produce more calculus than non-smokers. It is thought that irritation from the smoke results in an increased salivary flow rate. When saliva flow from the parotid gland, in particular, increases, the saliva produced has a higher pH and a raised concentration of calcium, resulting in increased precipitation of calcium phosphate. Calculus *per se* is relatively inert but it does have a rough surface which is plaque retentive, predisposing to periodontal problems in susceptible patients.[1]
- Epidemiological evidence suggests that smokers have higher plaque scores than non-smokers. This is not thought to be a direct effect of the smoking but is believed to be related to poorer plaque control.
- There is increasing evidence demonstrating that the incidence, prevalence and severity of periodontal disease seen in smokers is greater than in non-smokers (see Chapter 4).
- Vasoconstriction within the gingivae resulting from nicotine inhalation masks the important sign of BOP from the base of the pocket. Smokers must thus be examined carefully, otherwise the activity of periodontal disease may be underestimated.
- Vasoconstriction also results in reduced GCF flow. As discussed in Chapter 3, this contains many host-defence products, whose reduction is potentially damaging.
- It has been demonstrated that PMNLs derived from the gingival crevice in smokers show reduced chemotaxis, phagocytosis and migration rate (see Chapter 3). Reduced immune-inflammatory cell function is associated with aggressive forms of periodontitis.
- Smoking reduces the success of both surgical and non-surgical periodontal therapy. Nicotine is adsorbed onto the root surface in smokers and can result in fibroblast disorientation.

3. The dental team can play an important role in smoking cessation counselling and in helping patients who wish to reduce or stop smoking to achieve this. A great deal of information is available about how correctly to approach smoking cessation, but it is essential that patients know that quitting smoking will produce an oral health gain.

The question of whether certain forms of dental/periodontal therapy should be denied to smokers on the grounds that the likelihood of success is reduced is an emotive issue. Implant placement and guided tissue regeneration are often *not* offered to smokers, while conventional periodontal surgery may be. When a treatment is technically demanding and time-consuming for the clinician and costly for the patient, both may wish to maximise the chance of a successful outcome.

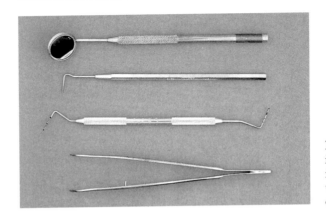

Fig 7-1 Photograph illustrating the basic instruments required to perform a clinical examination.

Alcohol consumption is also important from a periodontal standpoint owing to the effects of chronic alcoholism on liver function and hence blood clotting.

The Examination

The examination begins extra-orally and normally includes examination and, as required, testing of the function of the temporomandibular joints (TMJ), the orofacial musculature and regional lymph nodes. This is followed by a general intra-oral examination designed to look at the soft and hard tissues within the mouth as a whole. An examination kit designed to achieve this is shown in Fig 7-1, though each clinician will have their own preferred instruments.

The examination should include consideration of:
- Aesthetics. Is the patient content with this? If not, this may significantly affect the ultimate treatment plan.
- Gingival colour. Normal gingivae are conventionally described as being "pink", though within the wide limits of individual variation it can be difficult to ascribe a particular colour (see Chapter 5). Some inflamed areas are markedly red and are easily identified.
- Gingival contour. This is easier to see and there may be either swelling or recession/shrinkage. Swelling may be due to acute inflammation, in which case the gingivae are red and oedematous, or it may be caused by chronic

inflammation, in which case there is often much more fibrosis. In both situations plaque is the initiator of the pathology and the response to it can be exacerbated by other factors such as hormonal change. A number of medications have the undesired side-effect of gingival overgrowth, though not all patients are affected and the degree of involvement may vary greatly. The drugs in question include:

– phenytoin (e.g. Dilantin®), used to treat epilepsy
– calcium channel blockers (e.g. amlodipine), used to treat hypertension and angina
– ciclosporin, used post-transplantation to prevent organ rejection.

- Recession - This should be noted, and there may or may not be inflammation and/or pocketing at affected sites. Sometimes the problem is localised, but it may also be generalised. There are a number of different causes of recession, including past periodontal disease and a traumatic toothbrushing technique at sites with a relative lack of bone. Affected sites inevitably have root exposure, which may result in root caries and/or dentine hypersensitivity. If furcation areas are thus affected, loss of vitality may occur (see Chapter 8).

- Suppuration. The patient may report this directly or a bad taste may be described. Clinically it may be seen as a sinus, it may exude from beneath the gingival margin after a site has been probed, or it may be elicited by gentle massaging of the gingivae. The cause should always be identified, as treating the symptoms only (e.g. by prescribing antimicrobials) will not be successful in the medium to long term and is bad practice.

- Quality of restorations and their integrity. This is extremely significant when the periodontal condition is being assessed and when a treatment plan is to be devised. In short, defective margins act as plaque traps, and if subgingival are extremely difficult to clean. In susceptible patients the accumulated plaque will result in more periodontal disease and it is vital that both positive and negative defective margins on plastic restorations, crowns, bridges, implants, etc. are corrected in periodontitis-susceptible patients. Subgingival margins should also be noted and carefully probed.

- Removable appliances in the mouth should be examined for the same reasons as above. This would include orthodontic and prosthetic appliances.

- Caries if present should be noted including root caries. If there is a particular problem in this regard, a formal diet history should be elicited and a full preventive programme commenced.

- Occlusal examination is essential, to check for modifying factors of an underlying periodontitis (see Chapter 6). There may be evidence of tooth wear, reported TMJ problems (including pain, stiffness, trismus, deflected opening), tooth migration, increasing tooth mobility, or the presence

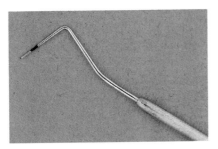

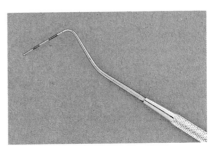

Fig 7-2 Photograph illustrating the basic points of a WHO-E (epidemiological)-type probe.

Fig 7-3 Photograph illustrating the basic points of a WHO-C (clinical)-type probe.

of a traumatic overbite. The occlusion should be checked clinically in all excursions and study models may also be necessary. If it is envisaged that the treatment plan will be complex, involving significant restorative work, occlusal assessment is mandatory.

Clearly, any abnormalities detected require further investigation and in any event all results, including those of negative findings should be carefully recorded and the notes legibly signed and dated.

Moving to the periodontal tissues, the following is a reasonable starting point. If the patient is new to you or has not been seen within the last year it is sensible to use the Basic Periodontal Examination (BPE) as recommended by the British Society of Periodontology (BSP). This is a rapid screening system which has been developed to aid the identification of "risk patients" with a significant periodontal problem, who therefore require a more detailed periodontal examination. It is not a quick alternative to a detailed examination in susceptible patients.

The BPE

The Probe

A special probe is required called the WHO (World Health Organization) probe. There are several variations upon the theme but the significant markings and measurements are as shown in Figs 7-2 and 7-3. The key elements include:

- a ball-end of 0.5mm diameter
- a coloured band extending from 3.5 to 5.5mm (WHO-E (epidemiological)-type probe)
- a second band is present in certain types of probe (WHO-C (clinical)-type probe) from 8.5 to11.5mm
- the target probing force should not exceed 0.2-0.25N (20-25g weight).

Division of the dentition
The dentition is divided into sextants as below (FDI notation):

17 – 14	13 – 23	24 – 27
47 – 44	43 – 33	34 – 37

If there are no teeth in a given sextant this is recorded as a cross in the chart (Fig 7-4). If only one tooth is present in a sextant, the sextant is recorded as having no teeth present as previous, and the single tooth is included in the adjacent sextant.

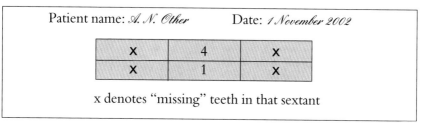

Patient name: *A. N. Other*   Date: *1 November 2002*

x	4	x
x	1	x

x denotes "missing" teeth in that sextant

Fig 7-4 Diagram of a BPE chart showing a cross in the sextants which have one or no teeth present.

How?
The probe tip is gently placed to the base of the pocket and the depth of insertion read against the colour coding. The total extent of the pocket should be explored conveniently by gently "walking" the probe around the entire gingival margin within each sextant. At least six points on each tooth should be examined: mesio-buccal, mid-buccal and disto-buccal and the corresponding lingual sites. For each sextant only one score/code is recorded and that is the highest encountered anywhere within it.

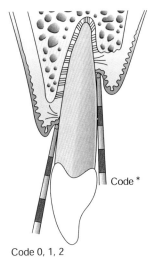

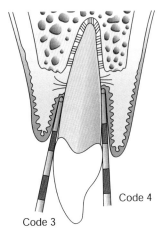

Fig 7-5 Diagram illustrating the BPE coding system in codes 0, 1, 2 + ★.

Fig 7-6 Diagram illustrating the BPE coding system in codes 3 and 4.

The scoring/coding system
This is best illustrated pictorially (Figs 7-5 and 7-6). In words:

Code 0 The coloured band on the probe is completely visible in the deepest pocket in the sextant. The gingival tissues are healthy, displaying no bleeding after gentle probing.

Code 1 The coloured band on the probe is completely visible in the deepest pocket in the sextant. There is no calculus and no plaque-retentive defective restoration margins are present. There is bleeding after gentle probing.

Code 2 The coloured band on the probe is completely visible in the deepest pocket in the sextant. Either, calculus (supragingival or subgingival) is present or there is a plaque-retentive/defective restoration margin.

Code 3 The coloured band on the probe is only partly visible in the deepest pocket in the sextant, indicating a PPD of 3.5-5.5mm.

Code 4 The coloured band on the probe is hidden in the deepest pocket in the sextant, indicating a pocket depth of ≥6mm.

Code ★ This denotes two special features:
- loss of attachment of ≥7mm or
- furcation involvement.

Recording the information
This is done using a box chart (Fig 7-7).

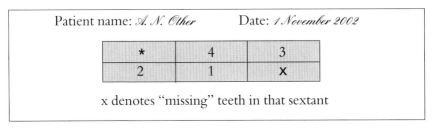

Patient name: *A. N. Other*   Date: *1 November 2002*

★	4	3
2	1	X

x denotes "missing" teeth in that sextant

Fig 7-7 Diagram illustrating a completed BPE chart.

Management according to score
The system suggests the following managements according to the score/code recorded:

Code 0: No treatment required
Code 1: Oral hygiene instruction (OHI)
Code 2: OHI plus calculus removal and/or correction of plaque-retentive restorative margins.

Patients with BPE scores of 0, 1 or 2 in all sextants should be screened again after one year.

Code 3: OHI plus scaling, restoration margin correction and root surface debridement (RSD), as required. Plaque and bleeding scores should be recorded at the start and finish of treatment. Pocket charts (see Chapter 8) should be recorded in sextants scoring code 3 at the finish of treatment. In addition, such sextants should have plaque, bleeding and pocket charts re-recorded at intervals of not more than one year along with BPE screening of the other sextants.

Code 4 or Code*: OHI plus scaling, margin correction and RSD as required. Surgery may be required later and referral to a specialist in periodontology should be considered. Plaque, bleeding and detailed pocket charts together with recordings of gingival recession, furcation involvement and any other relevant clinical details should be recorded at the start of treatment. Individual intra-oral radiographs of teeth which show furcation involvement or loss of attachment of ≥7mm should be taken (see Chapter 8). There should be a full re-examination after treatment to assess both the response to therapy and the subsequent potential requirement for further treatment, which may include surgery.

What are the Advantages and Disadvantages of the BPE?

As with all screening tests the BPE has benefits and disadvantages, and if it is to be used both correctly and to best advantage, knowledge of each is essential.

Advantages of the BPE
There are seven main ones:
1. It is a simple and rapid screening system which aids the identification of those individuals with significant periodontal disease who then require a much more detailed periodontal examination. However, the BPE is neither a short cut nor an alternative to a detailed examination in such cases. From a public health standpoint, identification of significantly affected persons should aid the targeting of scarce resources at those in most need.
2. The system is well recognised internationally, which aids communication of information across geographical boundaries.
3. The examination is both rapid and easy to complete.
4. The only equipment required is an appropriate probe and this is both readily available and inexpensive.
5. The system summarises the periodontal condition in a readily communicable form.
6. The system, as a whole, gives an indication of treatment appropriate to the codes assigned and suggests in some codes whether referral should be considered.
7. Perhaps because of a combination of the above factors, one of the best things about the BPE is that it encourages examination of the periodontal tissues in general practice. This is important for both clinicians and patients. Certainly in the current day, undiagnosed periodontal disease is one of the major causes of litigation in dentistry.

Disadvantages of the BPE

These are varied and include:

1. *Lack of detail within sextants.* This is an inevitable consequence of any hierarchical coding system, which requires only the highest score in any sextant to be recorded. The BPE provides no detail about either the number of affected sites or the severity of involvement, which can lead to confusion. For example, a sextant with one 6mm pocket would be assigned a code 4 while a sextant with generalised 5mm pockets would be assigned a code 3. Looking only at the codes one would assume that the periodontal condition was worse in the former rather than the latter case. Careful interpretation of results is thus vital.

2. *Lack of information on disease activity in all codes.* This is a consequence of a multi-faceted hierarchical coding system. The important sign of bleeding on probing from the base of the pocket is specifically referred to in only two codes – code 0 where it is not present and code 1 where it is. Once code 2 or higher is recorded, BOP becomes irrelevant to the index. Many people assume that this sign is present and part of codes 2, 3, 4 and ★ but this is not so – thus the system gives no indication of potential disease activity in these latter codes.

3. *Inability to provide information on loss of attachment* (LOA). This is an inherent consequence of the system as in all codes bar one assignation of code is based purely upon probing pocket depth. The exception is code ★ which implies either the presence of furcation involvement or LOA of ≥7mm. Lack of detail about LOA is a serious disadvantage as this important measurement gives vital information about disease experience.

4. *Inability to differentiate between true and false pockets.* This is a consequence again of having a system based almost exclusively on pocket depth measurements. This makes treatment planning difficult. For example, the treatment of choice for a 5mm *true pocket*, which exhibited BOP from the base of the pocket, would be to root plane the site (perform RSD). If the pocket was false, however, RSD would be entirely inappropriate, as new attachment onto the tooth crown could never occur.

5. *Lack of detail about furcation involvement.* Code ★ implies that furcation involvement may be present in a sextant but it does not give sufficient information. Ideally one should know which tooth is involved, which furcation(s) is/are involved and what the severity of the involvement is (see Chapter 8).

6. *BPE cannot be used for young individuals.* The gingival margin is often positioned coronal to the ACJ in young patients, as full clinical crown length maturation has not occurred. Using the BPE with its coding

system based on pocket depth would thus result in a tendency to over-estimate the code assigned.

7. *BPE cannot be used to monitor disease.* Although it is tempting to try, the BPE cannot be used to monitor disease due to the lack of detailed information available within sextants. Attempts at comparison using BPE codes only would be inherently meaningless.

8. *A special probe is required.* Although these are readily available, there is a capital cost involved in procuring them.

Is the BPE a Good Thing?

The million-dollar question! Basically, the answer is yes, provided the limitations are understood and the scores carefully interpreted. It does provide a quick and simple means of assessing whether significant periodontal disease is present in a mouth, and if so recommends detailed examination of the affected sextants. There is no excuse for not examining the periodontal condition of every patient, to determine those at risk of future attachment loss. For a minimal financial outlay and minimal time, BPE is practical and sensible.

Further Reading

Lindhe J, Karring T, Lang NP (Eds.) Clinical Periodontology and Implant Dentistry. 3rd ed. Copenhagen: Munksgaard, 1998.

Chapter 8
The Detailed Clinical Periodontal Examination

Aim

The purpose of this chapter is to outline the key stages involved in examining in detail patients identified as being susceptible to periodontitis.

Outcome

It is anticipated that having read this section, practitioners will understand the rationale for the individual measures recommended, and that they will be in a position to perform, record and interpret such assessments and produce appropriate treatment plans.

The Clinical Periodontal Examination

Having completed the extra-oral, general intra-oral and periodontal screening examinations, it should be apparent whether a detailed periodontal examination is necessary. If so, this will inevitably take a significant amount of time, but there are unfortunately no current alternatives. All sites to undergo a detailed examination need to be very carefully observed owing to the site-specific nature of the disease (see Chapter 5). No assumptions can be made about the mouth as a whole from a limited examination of only a few sites.

The detailed clinical examination comprises five separate parts and always precedes any radiological examination or other special tests. The information gained from this allows the clinician to decide on a logical basis whether additional tests are required and if so which ones. This ensures that only necessary tests are prescribed. The five components are:
- presence/absence of BOP
- PPD
- LOA
- furcation involvement
- mobility.

Lack of Bleeding on Probing from the Base of the Pocket

The first thing to be examined is whether there is or is not bleeding on probing from the base of the pockets.

Why?
Bleeding on probing from the base of the pocket is still regarded as the best individual clinical indicator of disease activity (Fig 8-1). Historically, BOP from the base of the pocket was thought to indicate the presence of active disease at that site at that time. Indeed this mantra recognised the concept of site specificity while acknowledging that disease is often episodic in nature. However, in the early 1990s, research demonstrated that only a maximum of 30% of sites exhibiting BOP from the base of pockets went on to lose attachment. It is thus more acceptable now to talk about lack of bleeding on probing from the base of the pocket, since we know that almost 100% of such sites in non-smokers will not progress to attachment loss. Whilst a lack of bleeding from the base of the pocket is associated with a lack of disease activity, the studies that demonstrated this did not take smoking habit into account. The absence of BOP from individual sites in current smokers cannot therefore be included in these interpretations.

How?
The assessment of BOP must be approached in a systematic manner ensuring that all sites are examined. It is thus important to get into a routine of performing this test in the same way each time, e.g. checking all buccal surfaces of the lower arch starting at, say, the lower left 7, progressing round the arch and then doing the equivalent for the upper arch. Once completed, this is repeated for the lingual/palatal surfaces. The examination is best accomplished by running a periodontal probe gently along the bases of appropriate gingival sulci and then checking to see whether bleeding occurs.

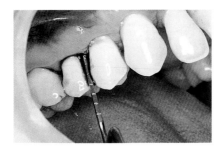

Fig 8-1 Photograph illustrating bleeding on probing from the base of the pocket.

It is important to keep the probe tip moving as applying point pressure may result in false positive results due to localised soft tissue penetration. Although any bleeding induced will be noticed at the gingival margin, it is essential that it is the tissues at the base of the pocket/gingival sulci that are tested. Sometimes the bleeding is immediate and profuse, while at other times it is delayed and scanty. It is suggested, therefore, that once a buccal or lingual quadrant has been completed, the clinician looks back along the quadrant sites tested so that delayed bleeding may be detected. The amount of bleeding produced is much less important than whether or not it occurs at all. It is because of this that many examiners choose to record BOP from sites qualitatively as being either present or absent. Although this may initially appear to be undervaluing detailed information, it does remove the problems of individual interpretation of more complex indices and the associated time involved.

Recording the Information
This may be done in a variety of ways, but perhaps the most succinct is via the type of chart shown in Fig 8-2. First, all missing teeth are deleted (illustrated by placing a horizontal line through the box representing the tooth) and those present are divided into 4 surfaces - buccal, lingual, mesial and distal. Presence or absence of BOP from the base of the pockets at each site is then noted and the appropiate segments coloured in – conventionally in red. Once completed, this format allows easy calculation of the percentage of sites affected and also allows pictorial representation of their distribution. This information is useful for both treatment planning at the beginning of therapy and at the re-evaluation phase, as well as being useful in patient motivation.

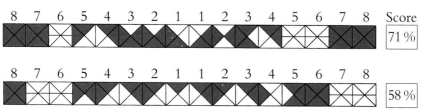

Patient name: *A. N. Other*   Date: *1 November 2002*

SITES WITH BLEEDING ON PROBING

| 8 | 7 | 6 | 5 | 4 | 3 | 2 | 1 | 1 | 2 | 3 | 4 | 5 | 6 | 7 | 8 | Score |

71 %

| 8 | 7 | 6 | 5 | 4 | 3 | 2 | 1 | 1 | 2 | 3 | 4 | 5 | 6 | 7 | 8 |

58 %

Fig 8-2 Photograph showing a completed bleeding chart.

Probing Pocket Depth (PPD)

Measurement of PPDs at as many sites as possible around the mouth is essential. Multiple site measurement is mandatory owing to the variation in periodontal disease experience seen within and between mouths.

Why?
In basic terms, if a pocket is ≤3mm, patients can keep the site clean using normal home-care methods. If pockets are deeper than this, patients cannot adequately clean them, resulting in an increased risk of continued destruction. One simple aim of periodontal therapy may therefore be regarded as reducing all PPDs to ≤3mm.

How?
PPD is the measurement from the gingival margin to the base of the pocket, when assessed by clinical probing (Chapter 1). It is measured using any one of a number of different periodontal probes (Fig 8-3) which all share the characteristics of having a blunt end to reduce the risk of tissue penetration and a series of markings along their length to facilitate the measurement process.

Recording the information
Some experienced clinicians find it quicker to record PPDs sequentially as buccal maxillary left quadrant, followed by palatal maxillary left quadrant, etc., and to circle sites that bleed on probing in red pen and sites of suppuration in blue/black pen. This clearly also provides six-sites-per-tooth assessment of BOP, but assumes the correct probing pressure has been used for bleeding scores. Whichever system is used depends on personal clinical preference. Should the clinician wish to have detailed records, a "double periodontal chart" such as that shown in Fig 8-4 is helpful. Specific details of how to complete this type of pocket chart are given later in this chapter.

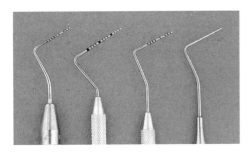

Fig 8-3 Photograph illustrating several types of periodontal probe.

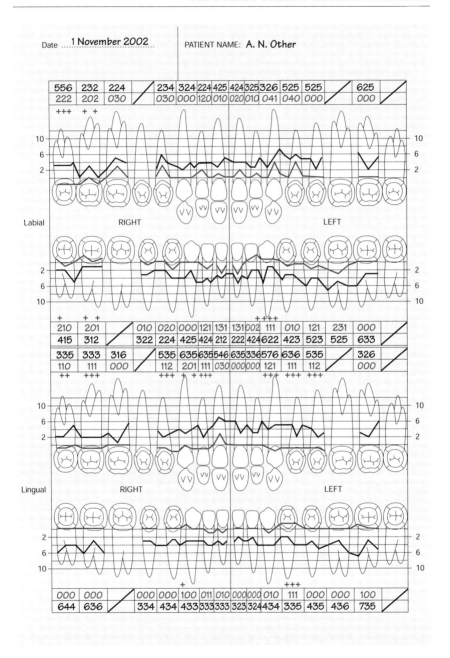

Fig 8-4 Completed "double periodontal chart".

115

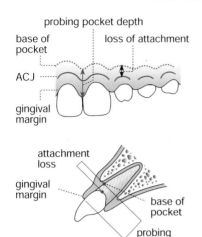

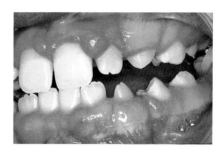

Fig 8-5 Photograph of gingival enlargement and diagram to show how both LOA and PPD would be measured. In this case, the PPD is greater than the LOA.

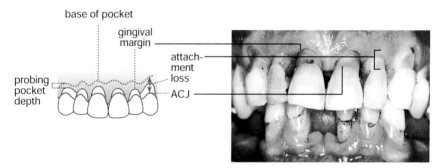

Fig 8-6 Photograph of gingival recession and diagram showing how both LOA and PPD would be measured. In this case, the PPD is less than the LOA.

LOA

Measurement of LOA at as many sites as possible around the mouth is important.

Why?
LOA is a measure of the sum total of periodontal destruction experienced at a particular site since the tooth erupted. It does not, however, provide information about the number of episodes of disease that have taken place or when they occurred. In terms of examination, diagnosis and treatment planning, it should be regarded as the background upon which the current detail of pocket depth should be placed.

How?
LOA is the measurement from the amelo-cemental junction (ACJ) to the base of the pocket.

Significance?
Usually pocket depth and LOA are different – only if the gingival margin lies at the ACJ will they be the same. In sites with gingival enlargement (Fig 8-5) pocket depth will exceed LOA and reliance upon pocket depth alone as an indicator of past disease experience will lead to over-estimation. The opposite is true in sites exhibiting recession/shrinkage (Fig 8-6), where using pocket depth alone would lead the observer to under-estimate disease experience.

Recording the information
The "double periodontal chart" discussed below is a good means of identifying this information.

Furcation Involvement

This refers to the recognition of horizontal loss of support in the areas where the roots of multi-rooted teeth converge.

Significance?
It is important to check for furcation involvement as this may reduce the prognosis for a tooth for two reasons:
1. The involved sites are difficult for both the clinician and the patient to gain access to and thus to clean. Thus controlling disease and preventing recurrence at such sites is less likely.

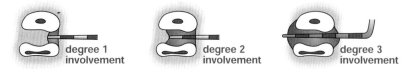

Fig 8-7 Diagram illustrating the different degrees of furcation involvement.

2. Loss of vitality of the involved tooth/teeth may occur. This happens because accessory canals running from the pulp chamber to the furcation area act as a conduit for bacteria and their products. Assault on the pulp in this manner is often symptom free.

Detection?
Clinical examination is essential and is facilitated using a curved furcation probe to measure horizontal loss of support. The teeth to check are as follows:
• *Maxillary first premolars* usually have a buccal and a palatal root so clinical detection of furcation involvement should be from both the mesial and distal aspects.
• *Mandibular molars* usually have one mesial and one distal root so clinical detection of furcation involvement should be from both the buccal and lingual aspects.
• *Maxillary molars* usually have one large palatal root and both a mesio-buccal and a disto-buccal root. Clinical examination to detect the presence of furcation involvement in these teeth should be from the buccal aspect between the two buccal roots, from the mesial aspect (approaching from the palatal side of the embrasure) and from the distal aspect (which may be approached from either side of the embrasure).

Grading the severity of furcation involvement
This is important as the definitive treatment of a furcation lesion depends upon the degree of involvement. There are many classification systems but that suggested by Hamp *et al.* (1975) is to be commended for its simplicity and pragmatism. In this system (Fig 8-7):
Degree 1 = horizontal loss of periodontal support not exceeding one-third of the bucco-lingual width of the tooth.
Degree 2 = horizontal loss of periodontal support exceeding one-third of the width of the tooth, but not encompassing the total width of the furcation area.

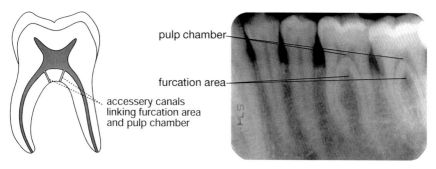

Fig 8-8 Radiograph illustrating the proximity of the pulp chamber to the furcation area, and a diagram showing stylised accessory canals linking the two.

Degree 3 = horizontal "through and through" destruction of the periodontal tissues in the furcation area.

Reporting furcation involvement
The clinician should always note which tooth has furcation involvement, which furcation(s) is/are affected and the degree of involvement present at each affected site.

Differential diagnosis
In addition to being caused by periodontal disease, a lesion in the furcation area may be associated with problems originating from the root canal or be the result of occlusal overload. Treatment should not therefore be initiated until a definitive diagnosis has been made for the lesion.

Vitality testing
It is advisable to "vitality-test" all teeth displaying furcation involvement. This is necessary because loss of vitality can occur in such teeth – often without symptoms. This may happen owing to infection of accessory canals (see Fig 8-8). Toxins from plaque lying in the furcation area have a very short distance to travel through these canals to reach, and ultimately render nonvital, pulpal tissue in one or more canals. Naturally, if this occurs, either root canal therapy or extraction of the affected tooth will be necessary.

Tooth Mobility

Tooth mobility should be checked for all teeth and is important for monitoring changes in the degree of mobility from visit to visit and also to inform treatment planning. Clearly, if a tooth displays degree 2 mobility and has done so for a period of years, this is of less concern than one which now has this degree of mobility but 3 months earlier exhibited no mobility. In general, the higher the mobility the poorer the prognosis.

How?
The handles of two hand instruments are used, and pressure is placed on the crown of the tooth to be tested, alternately from the buccal and lingual aspects and also vertically down the long axis of the tooth.

Grading of tooth mobility
Unfortunately, grading is rather subjective, but using a system is better than using very imprecise terms such as "slightly" or "moderately", as these have different meanings to different people. There are a number of choices but a simple and practical one is documented below:

Degree 0 = no detectable movement/physiological mobility (classically up to 0.2mm).

Degree 1 = mobility of the crown of the tooth 0.2-1mm in the horizontal direction.

Degree 2 = mobility of the crown of the tooth >1mm in the horizontal direction.

Degree 3 = mobility of the crown in both the horizontal and vertical planes.

Causes of tooth mobility
This should always be considered in addition to examining the degree of involvement, because effective treatment depends upon an accurate diagnosis of the cause(s). There are three main causes, which may apply singly or in any combination:

    trauma – either direct blunt trauma or occlusal trauma
    periapical disease
    periodontal disease leading to loss of support.

Recording the information
This is best done using a chart such as that in Fig 8-9. Each box represents a particular tooth and after deletion of missing teeth the mobility score, graded from 0 to 3, as above, is placed within the appropriate box.

Mobility

Patient name: *A. N. Another*　　Date: *1 November 2002*

8	7	6	5	4	3	2	1	1	2	3	4	5	6	7	8
1	2	—	2	1	O	O	1	1	O	O	1	—	—	1	1

8	7	6	5	4	3	2	1	1	2	3	4	5	6	7	8
2	—	—	1	O	O	O	O	1	O	O	O	1	1	—	—

Fig 8-9 Completed mobility chart.

Recording a "Double Periodontal Chart"

Why?
Initial charts provide a record of the baseline periodontal status and subsequent charts demonstrate how measurements change at specific sites over time with treatment.

How?
This exercise requires the presence of a chairside assistant to record the data. The procedure is as follows:

1. Record all missing teeth and delete them from the chart.
2. Record the gingival margin measurement (usually recorded in red). Ensure that the assistant knows exactly where you are starting from, e.g. buccal upper left 7, and then measure the distance in millimetres (mm) from the gingival margin to the ACJ using a suitable banded probe. The ACJ may be detected either visually or by touch. The "mm" reading from the probe is recorded as a plus if the gingival margin lies coronal to the ACJ (e.g. +2: Fig 8-10), while it is recorded as simply the number of mm (with neither a plus nor a minus) when the gingival margin lies apical to the ACJ (Fig 8-11).
3. Three measurements are recorded for the buccal surface of each tooth (i.e. disto-buccal, mid-buccal and mesio-buccal) and the appropriate results are placed in the corresponding boxes on the chart (Fig 8-12).
4. The recording occurs in a systematic manner to ensure that no teeth or sites are missed. However, it is possible that mistakes can unwittingly occur and it is advisable on reaching the midline to state this. Should there be a discrepancy between the dentist and assistant, then it will become clear at this stage and may be rectified immediately.

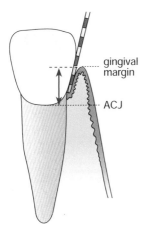

Fig 8-10 Diagram illustrating a periodontal probe being used to measure the distance of the gingival margin to the ACJ in a site of gingival enlargement. The measurement in mm is recorded as a "plus" score.

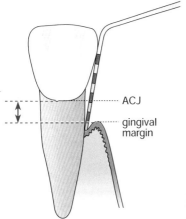

Fig 8-11 Diagram as above except in a site exhibiting gingival recession. The measurement is given in mm only with no "plus" or "minus" designation.

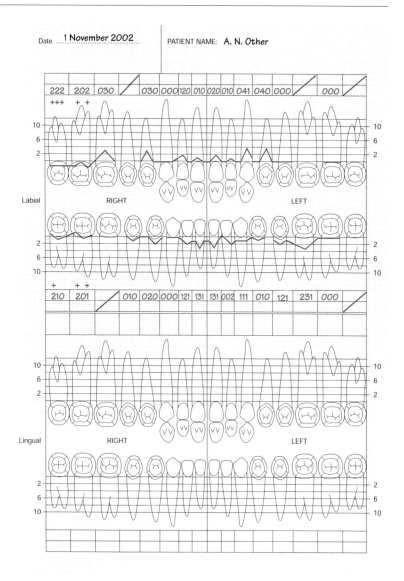

Fig 8-12 Partially completed "double periodontal chart" showing missing teeth ▨ and the measurements in mm from the ACJ to the gingival margin on the buccal/labial surfaces of the teeth. The measurements are then transferred to lie on top of the drawings of the teeth in the correct position and the red line representing the position of the gingival margin is generated by joining them up.

5. Once the buccal surfaces of both arches have been examined, recording of data from the palatal/lingual surfaces may proceed. This is completed in the same systematic manner.

6. The PPD measurements are then recorded (usually in blue). This is done using the probe to measure the distance from the gingival margin to the base of the pocket. As described above, this data is retrieved from a total of six sites around each tooth – three buccal and three lingual/palatal.

7. Once all the appropriate figures have been filled in on the chart boxes the "whole mouth picture" becomes clear. Some clinicians prefer to join all the points drawn on the chart, to provide a rough visual summary. In this situation, the gingival margin line is usually completed first and by convention is depicted in red. The line representing the base of the pocket is then drawn in (by convention, in blue) by measuring the distance recorded for pocket depth from the red line representing the gingival margin (Fig 8-4). However, it is important to recognise that such lines represent an estimate of the attachment contour between recorded points and are not truly accurate.

Advantages
The completed chart allows examination of the following at six points around each tooth in the whole mouth.

1. PPD measured from the gingival margin to the base of the pocket.
2. LOA measured from the ACJ to the base of the pocket.
3. The pattern of both PPD and LOA throughout the mouth. The latter is very helpful in reaching a periodontal diagnosis as both severity and distribution are exhibited.
4. The presence and location of gingival enlargement/recession is demonstrated (the distance from the ACJ to the gingival margin).

Disadvantages
There are two main disadvantages of double periodontal charts in addition to the assumptions made when the measured points are linked using a line:

1. There is an inherent risk of inaccuracy with all measurements based on probing, which can lead to under- or overestimation of measurements. This is discussed below.
2. The procedure takes considerable time, though this reduces with experience. In any case this has to be weighed against the information gained.

Many computerised software programs facilitate periodontal charting in practice, but many are limited and do not allow the recording of attachment loss.

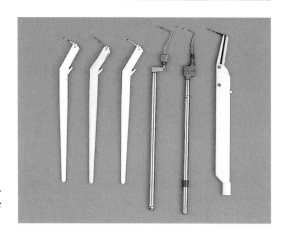

Fig 8-13 Photograph of a selection of pressure-sensitive probes.

Errors Associated with Manual Probing

The measurements produced are clearly operator sensitive and several factors affect the accuracy of the results gained. These include:

1. *The probing force applied.* Ideally this should be around 0.2-0.25N (20-25g weight for typical probes), though it is known that large variations arise in the probing force applied even by the same operator at different sites in the same mouth. Excessive force will result in penetration of the tissues at the base of the pocket and thus overestimation of the true probing pocket depth occurs. Alternatively, application of too little force may mean that the base of the pocket is not reached and pocket depth underestimation may result. Pressure-sensitive probes have been developed which do not permit the application of forces greater than a set maximum (Fig 8-13). They do not, however, prevent variation in probing forces which may be applied below that maximum.

2. *The size and shape of the probe.* A thick or broad probe will not be able to negotiate a narrow or tortuous pocket and may result in underestimation of probing depth. Equally, a sharp probe, even applied at appropriate pressure, could easily penetrate the soft tissues at the base of the pocket and result in overestimation.

3. *The inflammatory state of the tissues.* If the base of the pocket is inflamed, a high percentage of the collagen in the connective tissue at the pocket base is lost. This means that the tissue has poor resistance and application of a probe, even at normal forces, will often result in tissue penetration and thus overestimation of pocket depth measurements.

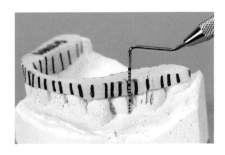

Fig 8-14 Photograph of a stent.

4. *The presence of calculus, over-contoured restorations, bulbous crowns and un-favourable root morphology.* Calculus is very common when patients first present for treatment and these deposits may prevent negotiation of the probe to the base of the pocket. This results in underestimation of pocket depths introducing errors at the time of the initial examination, and also giving the impression of apparent deepening of pockets after therapy, when these deposits have been removed facilitating access to the base of the pocket. Presence of over-contoured restorations, bulbous crowns and very curved roots also prevent adequate negotiation of the pocket by the probe, with similar resultant potential problems.

5. *The angle of the probe.* If the probe is placed at an angle other than parallel to the long axis of the tooth this may result in overestimation of the pocket depth.

6. *Variation in probing position.* If sequential measurements are made and the probe is not introduced at precisely the same point each time, comparative measurements are very difficult. In clinical trials, occlusal stents are used to reduce this source of error (see Fig 8-14).

7. *Clarity of banding on the probe.* Making measurements is difficult if the bands on the probe are indistinct and difficult to interpret, which may result in operator errors.

8. *Patient tolerance.* This varies, and if it is low, reaching the base of the pocket to make measurements can be difficult if not impossible. If this occurs, charting may have to be done by sextant/quadrant after administration of local anaesthetic, prior to commencing treatment of that area.

Choice of probe

Electronic probes (Fig 8-15) as well as manual probes are now available. The former are certainly capable of greater accuracy of measurement (up to 0.1mm), but the reproducibility of electronic probing is no greater than that with manual probing (Fig 8-16). In general, electronic probes have two main advantages:

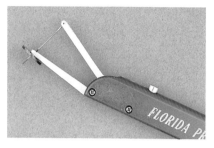

Fig 8-15 Florida electronic probe, with constant force and automated recording by foot pedal.

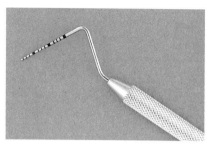

Fig 8-16 University of North Carolina (UNC-15) probe.

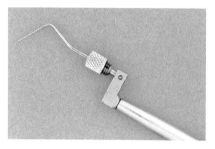

Fig 8-17 Brodontic manual constant force probe.

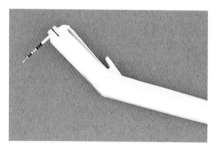

Fig 8-18 TPS plastic constant force probe.

- they permit objective data recording, which is not dependent upon operator eyesight
- there is a constant probing force – usually standardised at 0.25N.

Electronic probes are expensive, however, and manual probes which use a constant force (Fig 8-17) and a standard tip diameter (0.5mm) with clearer banding are now available at considerably less cost. In addition, some clinicians believe that plastic probes (Fig 8-18) more readily follow tortuous pockets and unfavourable contours. On the downside, it must be added that plastic probes:

- provide less tactile feedback
- deform more easily
- can be an expensive option as the cost is recurrent because they are disposable.

Which probe you choose is entirely up to you!

What about Plaque Scores?

Plaque is the initiator of periodontal inflammation, but by itself the plaque score gives no information about periodontal disease experience. As discussed in Chapter 4, patients with low susceptibility to periodontal disease may display high plaque scores, while exhibiting little evidence of destructive disease. The opposite can occur also. This does not mean that plaque scores are irrelevant – indeed they play an important part in treatment planning, particularly for highly susceptible individuals. In isolation, however, they tell us nothing about the disease to be found in a mouth, and it is important to recognise that a majority of patients will clean their teeth immediately prior to a dental appointment.

Further Reading

Galgutt PN, Dowsett SA, Kowolik MJ (Eds.) Periodontics: Current Concepts and Treatment Strategies. London: Martin Dunitz, 2001: Chapter 8.

Hamp SE, Nyman S, Lindhe J. Periodontal treatment of multirooted teeth (results after five years) J Clin Periodontol 1975;7:126.

Chapter 9
Radiographic Examination and Special Tests

Aim

This chapter aims to outline the indications and contraindications for using special tests during a detailed periodontal assessment. Advantages and disadvantages of different types of radiographic examinations are discussed alongside other special tests.

Outcome

The outcome of reading this chapter will be that the practitioner should be clear about which radiographs to take in which situations, and how to interpret results in terms of a periodontal assessment and document radiographic reports.

The clinical examination precedes any other "hands-on" investigation and determines whether, and if so which, special tests need to be performed. They are not always required.

The Radiographic Examination

Radiographs are used to provide information largely about hard tissues and are recommended only when such data provides positive added value to that already held. There are a number of points to consider:

1. A balance needs to be struck for individual patients in individual circumstances between the advantages of the additional diagnostic yield gained from taking radiographs and the potential disadvantages of exposure to radiation.
2. If radiographs are to be taken, the clinician must choose films that will provide the highest diagnostic yield for the least possible radiation.
3. There should be a signed and dated radiographic report in the notes pertaining to all radiographs taken.
4. Should there be difficulty in interpretation of radiographs an opinion should be sought from a radiologist and a written report requested.

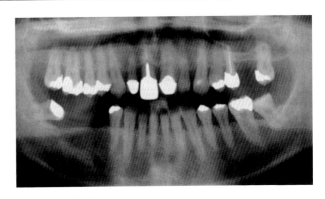

Fig 9-1
DPT radiograph.

Choice of Techniques

Fast (E- or F-speed) films and narrowly collimated X-ray beams should be used to decrease radiation doses as much as possible. Three types of film are routinely used in conventional dental radiography: dental panoramic tomograms, bitewings and periapicals.

Dental panoramic tomograms (DPT)
Dental panoramic tomograms give a general overall view of the mouth, permitting a general examination of the teeth and jaws. An example is shown in Fig 9-1. Unfortunately, distortions in the horizontal plane are frequently found. In particular, DPTs are less clear around the lower anterior region owing to both superimposition of the cervical spine and distortion in this area. The quality of DPTs has improved greatly in recent years, though most clinicians would accept that the image quality is not yet as good as that from intra-oral films. The radiation dose from a DPT is, however, significantly less than that from full-mouth intra-oral radiographs.

Bitewings
Bitewings can be used in two planes – vertical or horizontal. Horizontal bitewings (Fig 9-2) are often taken in general practice to look for interproximal caries and can also be used to look for marginal bone loss in mild to moderate periodontal disease. In such circumstances, a single film will show the bone crest in both arches and the radiation dose is relatively small. This type of film does not, however, show the periapical tissues and sometimes the furcation areas are also not visible. Compared to horizontal bitewings, vertical bitewings show a greater percentage of the teeth being filmed though fewer teeth are displayed on each one. Vertical bitewings may

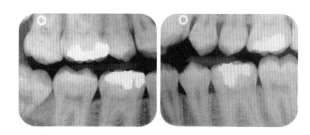

Fig 9-2
Horizontal bitewing
radiographs.

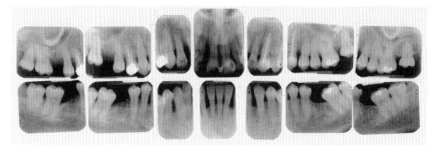

Fig 9-3 Full-mouth periapical radiographs.

be used to display the marginal bone crest and the furcation areas of the filmed teeth though often the periapical areas are not visible.

Periapicals
Periapicals are the films of choice when the finest detail is required and imaging of the apical and periapical tissues is necessary. Periapical views (PAs) will give the most information possible about individual teeth and their support – including the furcation and periapical areas – though if full mouth films are taken there is an increased radiation dose for the patient compared to taking a single DPT. The best results are obtained using a long cone paralleling technique with the use of film holders, as this produces the least distortion. The bisecting-angle technique should be avoided because it results in underestimation of bone loss. If the clinician wishes to assess the root length and shape then the PA is the film of choice. A set of full-mouth periapical films is shown in Fig 9-3. In order to minimise radiation dosage it would be unusual to repeat full-mouth periapicals within two years. It may, however, prove necessary to repeat individual periapical films within this time if particular problems arise, though there must be a compelling clinical reason to do so.

The newer technique of digital radiography is becoming more widely available and presents a number of advantages, not least because it reduces the radiation exposure for the patient. In addition, it permits varied manipulation of the images produced and facilitates the assessment of specific measurements. Digital subtraction radiography (DSR), in particular, is useful for highlighting small changes in bone loss over time. For accurate comparisons using this technique, it is essential that the films being examined have been taken in precisely the same way. The use of film holders and stents, etc. is required to achieve this, which inherently makes the physical process rather more complicated and time-consuming. Switching to this technology involves considerable capital outlay but it seems to be where the future lies.

Which Films to Take

There are no fixed rules for this but Table 9-1 is a guide.

Advantages of Radiographs

Radiographs clearly facilitate visualisation of hard tissues, thereby enabling examination of root and bone anatomy and pathology, prior to preparation of the radiological report.

The Radiological Report

The rate of change is often significant so documentation of radiological findings is important as it permits longitudinal examination of features over time. When preparing the report there should be consideration of the following points. Negative findings should also be included.

1. Charting of the teeth present.
2. Bone loss. Consideration of this is important in periodontal diagnosis. It should be remembered, however, that only interproximal bone can be examined with any clarity from radiographs, as the high radio-density of the teeth themselves prevents visualisation of bone overlying them. Three aspects of bone loss should be considered: severity, pattern and distribution.

The severity
In the past this used to be calculated as a simple linear measurement in millimetres (mm) from the ACJ to the bone crest (Fig 9-4). This was subsequently judged to be an inadequate method, for a number of reasons. First, it took no cognisance of the original root length. This is significant as a 5mm linear loss of bone in someone with short roots is much more

Table 9-1 **Which films to take – a suggestion**

Disease	Distribution	Severity	Radiograph
Gingivitis			None
Periodontitis	generalised	mild (LOA ≤ 3mm)	DPT
		moderate (LOA >3mm but <5mm)	DPT and supplemental films of localised areas (e.g. furcation involvements) using PAs or vertical bitewings
		severe (LOA >5mm)	periapicals of standing teeth or DPT if considering clearance
Periodontitis	localised – posterior teeth only affected	mild	horizontal bite-wings
		moderate	vertical bite-wings
		severe	periapicals of affected teeth or DPT initially ± supplemental PAs
Periodontitis	localised – anterior teeth only affected	mild	periapicals of affected teeth or DPT initially ± supplemental PAs
		moderate	as above
		severe	as above
Periodontitis	localised involving anterior and posterior teeth	mild	DPT
		moderate	DPT initially ± vertical bitewings for posteriors ± PAs for anterior teeth
		severe	periapicals of standing teeth or DPT initially ± supplemental PAs

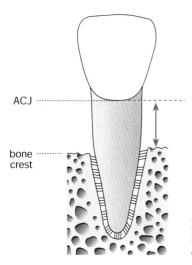

ACJ

bone
crest

Fig 9-4 Diagram to illustrate old-style linear measurement of bone loss from ACJ to bone crest.

serious than the same loss occurring in someone with much longer roots. Secondly, it was recognised that a radiograph presents only an image of a tooth or teeth and that this image may be foreshortened or lengthened. Direct measurements taken from a radiograph may thus be similarly distorted, making any results gained questionable at best. The solution is to look at the percentage of the root no longer covered by bone, as this proportion will not change irrespective of foreshortening or lengthening. The measurement of bone loss is thus represented by the formula:

$$\frac{ACJ - bone\ crest\ (in\ mm)}{ACJ - root\ apex\ (in\ mm)} \times 100$$

Thus, for example, a surface may show 50% bone loss.

The pattern
Two main patterns of bone loss are discernible. The first is horizontal bone loss (Fig 9-5), which occurs when the interproximal bone crest is lost essentially evenly between the teeth being examined. This pattern of bone loss is associated with supra-bony true pockets, in which the base of the pocket lies coronal to the bone crest (Fig 9-6). The other is vertical/angular bone loss. The terms "vertical" and "angular" are often used interchangeably and mean the same thing (Fig 9-7). Vertical bone loss occurs when more bone is lost on one side of the interdental bone crest than

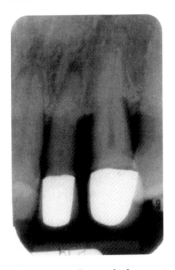

Fig 9-5 Radiograph demonstrating horizontal bone loss.

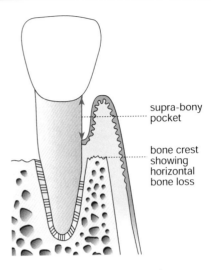

Fig 9-6 Diagram representing suprabony pocketing.

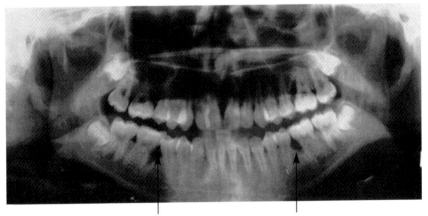

Vertical/angular bone defects

Fig 9-7 Radiograph demonstrating vertical/angular bone loss.

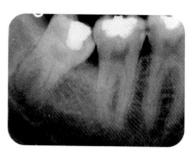

Fig 9-9 Radiograph demonstrating caries between the first and second molars and on the third molar.

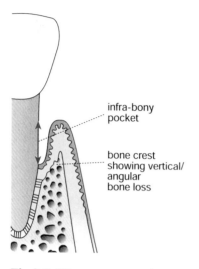

infra-bony pocket

bone crest showing vertical/angular bone loss

Fig 9-8 Diagram representing infra-bony pocketing.

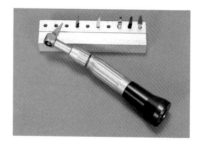

Fig 9-10 Photograph of reciprocating handpiece with inserts.

on the other. This pattern is associated with infra-bony true pockets, in which the base of the pocket lies within the bone defect created (Fig 9-8).

The distribution

This should be noted as being either localised or generalised. One way of defining this would be to say that if ≤ 30% of sites are affected the condition would be described as being localised and if >30% of sites are affected it would be considered to be generalised (see Chapter 6).

3. Caries. This should be noted whether "primary" or "secondary" and corrective measures should be part of the subsequent treatment plan (Fig 9-9).

4. Overhanging restorations. These should be noted and their removal or recontouring should be quickly effected. They are obvious plaque traps and there is no point in embarking upon periodontal therapy if they remain. This is particularly true for patients with a high susceptibility to periodontal disease. Sometimes overhangs may be removed by use of fin-

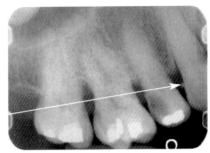

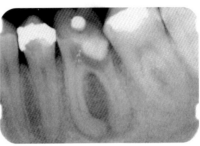

Fig 9-11 Radiograph demonstrating calculus.

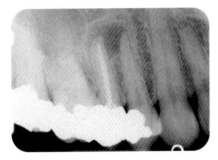

Fig 9-12 Radiographs demonstrating periapical areas.

ishing strips, finishing burs, reciprocating handpieces (Fig 9-10) or even via the use of an ultrasonic scaler. If none of these options proves effective, then replacement of the affected restorations is required.

5. Calculus. Two factors determine whether calculus is seen on a radiograph.

Degree of mineralisation
The degree of mineralisation varies and there is a minimum threshold below which it will not be visible on radiographs.

Location
Calculus on the tooth will usually only be visible if it is located in the interproximal regions. This is because the teeth are so radio-dense that they obscure superimposed calculus.

The interpretation of radiographs with regard to calculus must therefore be carefully considered. If calculus is seen on a film it is definitely present. If it is not visible on a film then it may be present, but in another location, or may be too poorly mineralised to permit visualisation (Fig 9-11).

6. Periapical pathology. This must be identified and should, if possible, be compared with previous films to provide an indication of how long a

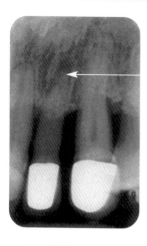

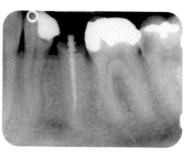

Fig 9-13 Radiograph demonstrating loss of the lamina dura.

Fig 9-14 Radiograph demonstrating the mental foramen lying close to the lower premolars.

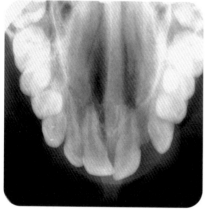

Fig 9-15 Radiograph demonstrating the incisive foramen lying close to the apices of the upper central incisors.

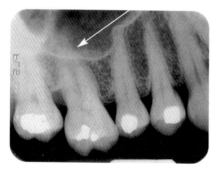

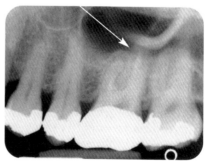

Fig 9-16 Radiographs demonstrating apparent periapical areas due to superimposition of maxillary roots over antral air space.

138

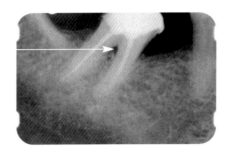

Fig 9-17 Radiograph demonstrating an arrow-head lesion.

lesion has been present and whether it is enlarging or declining in size. Periapical areas may be an incidental finding on a radiograph or the film may confirm suspicions from the clinical examination (Fig 9-12). The first sign of this type of lesion occurring is loss of the continuity of the lamina dura (Fig 9-13), and if this is observed the tooth involved should have its vitality checked and the occlusion should be similarly examined. Should a tooth turn out to be both periodontally and endodontically involved – a true combined lesion – the endodontic treatment should always precede periodontal therapy. This is necessary as the degenerating remains of a necrotic pulp release toxins through the apex, through lateral and accessory canals and possibly through dentinal tubules. Such toxins entering into the periodontal ligament will prevent healing of the site even if periodontal therapy is undertaken. The first step is thus to remove the reservoir of toxins from within the tooth. It is also important not to confuse normal anatomical features with periapical disease. Commonly, problems arise with apparent superimposition of the mental foramen upon the lower premolars (Fig 9-14), the incisive foramen upon the upper central incisors (Fig 9-15) and the maxillary sinus upon the upper posterior teeth sometimes giving the appearance of periapical areas (Fig 9-16).

7. Suggestion of furcation involvement. The diagnosis of furcation involvement is always clinical (see Chapter 8), though the presence of an arrow-head lesion (Fig 9-17) on a radiograph should alert the clinician to the possibility and ensure that clinical re-examination occurs.

8. Presence of root fractures and other pathology. Radiographs may demonstrate the presence of a root fracture. Any present should be noted and if necessary expert advice sought for specific diagnosis.

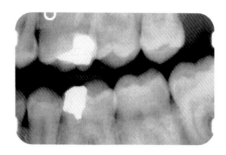

Fig 9-18 Radiograph demonstrating tooth-on-tooth superimposition.

Two bone crests seen

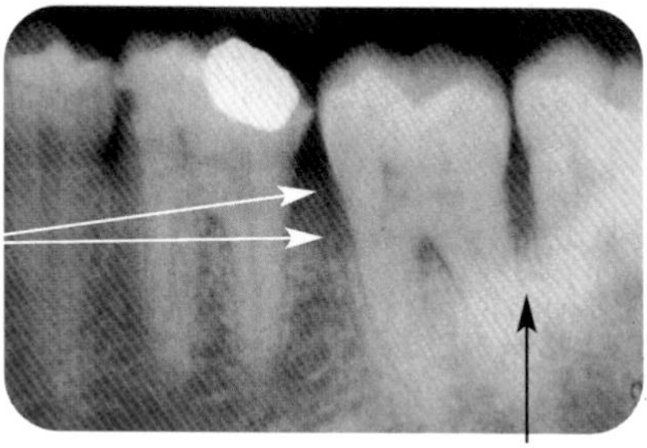

Fig 9-19 Radiograph demonstrating bone-on-bone superimposition.

Superimposition by external oblique ridge of mandible

Disadvantages of Radiographs

The disadvantages of radiographs must be understood if correct interpretation of the scrutinised films is to occur. These include:

1. Superimposition. A radiograph converts a three-dimensional object into a two-dimensional image and this inevitably results in superimposition. This occurs in three ways: tooth-on-tooth superimposition, tooth-on-bone superimposition and bone-on-bone superimposition.

   Tooth-on-tooth superimposition (Fig 9-18). This means that it is not possible to look at all surfaces of the teeth involved, as their images lie at least partially on top of one another.

   Tooth-on-bone superimposition occurs all around the mouth. This is the reason that bone is visible only interproximally as the teeth being so radiodense do not permit clear visualisation of the bone overlying them.

   Bone-on-bone superimposition (Fig 9-19) occurs because the buccal and lingual plates of bone do not necessarily resorb evenly and when superimposed a double shadow of bone may be seen. In addition, if cortical bone remains intact the extent of a defect lying within these walls may be masked radiographically by the intact buccal or lingual bone plates. However, changes in bone density may be seen in such sites if the clinician examines the sites very carefully.

2. Underestimation of bone loss. This means that if a radiograph of a site is compared with surgical exposure of the same site, the radiograph would usually underestimate the bone loss. It is important to remember this when deciding whether to retain and attempt to treat teeth with severe periodontal involvement.

3. No indication of disease activity. Lack of disease activity is indicated by a lack of bleeding from the base of the pockets after gentle probing. Radiographs give no indication of this clinical sign as they indicate only historical disease experience in hard tissues.

4. No indication of pocket depth, loss of attachment or mobility. All these are assessed clinically and radiographs have no role in this process.

5. Limited indication of the history of the disease. Radiographs give a snapshot image of the hard tissues at the time the films were taken. It is thus not possible by looking at one set of films to know either for how long any disease has been progressing or how many episodes of disease have taken place. This means that it is not possible to ascertain whether destruction seen on a film took place some time ago and the disease has now "burnt out", or whether it all happened recently.

6. Assessment of small changes over time is difficult. Even with sequential conventional radiographic assessment, detecting small changes in bone loss is difficult. This problem may be at least partly overcome by use of DSR.

7. Radiation of the patient. Radiation is the biological cost, paid by the patient, for the diagnostic yield that the films provide. It is because of this that films must only be taken when there is a clear clinical indication to do so. The radiation dose used must be the minimum possible to obtain the information needed and the films taken must be fully reported to maximise the information gain.

With So Many Disadvantages Are Radiographs a Good Thing?

The answer to this is a qualified yes, though the clinician has a duty to weigh up both the need for radiographs and the numbers and types required very carefully.

Special Tests

Special tests are required by relatively few patients but are essential for some. The most common are:

1. Blood tests. There are many different types of blood test, designed to investigate a particular aspect of biological importance. Blood tests should

141

be considered in patients with severe disease which is not commensurate with their plaque levels. This becomes even more important if the response to treatment is poor despite clear evidence of co-operation with instructions given. Blood screening should also be considered if patients with periodontal disease are systemically unwell. It is possible that the periodontal destruction exhibited may be accounted for, at least in part, by systemic factors. The most common blood tests are detailed below.

The full blood count (FBC) – this provides basic information on blood cell and platelet numbers and their relative levels. This may highlight, for example, the presence of a neutropenia, a condition reported to be associated with gingival ulceration and increased risk of periodontal damage.

A differential white blood cell count – this is obtained routinely from a FBC, and can help to eliminate conditions such as leukaemia. Increased leucocyte numbers (leucocytosis) are associated with significant periodontitis, as the body mounts an immune response to the relevant pathogens.

Blood films – are tests for blood cell size and shape. Results from FBCs will provide information on increased or decreased cell size (macro-/microcytosis) as seen in B12/folate and iron deficiency respectively. However, subtle changes of cell form require a haematologist to view cells microscopically, rather than relying on automated cell counters (haemocytometers) for FBCs. Defects of platelet function, for example, will not be detected by a FBC, as platelet numbers may be normal.

Blood glucose testing is performed if diabetes is suspected, though if the results are unclear, glycated haemoglobin levels may be required (see Chapter 4).

Immunology – Various levels of immunoglobulin and complement, as well as so-called acute-phase proteins (produced by the liver), provide non-specific indications of infective load. However, the investigation of desquamative gingivitis relies upon identifying auto-antibodies to epithelial basement membrane or intercellular cement (cadherin molecules), using indirect immunofluorescence. PMNL-function tests may also help identify underlying defects of neutrophil function in aggressive periodontitis, but most immunological assays are best performed in specialist centres.

2. Vitality testing. This is essential if there is a possibility that vitality may have been lost in a tooth. The question may arise because a tooth becomes darkened, because evidence of periapical radiolucency is seen on radiographs, or because the clinical presentation, including the presence of furcation involvement, otherwise suggests it. It is important to know if loss of vitality has occurred because the outcome will inevitably change a treat-

Fig 9-20 Using a GP point to locate the source of infection.

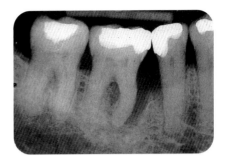

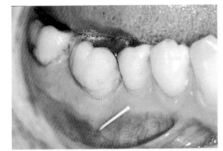

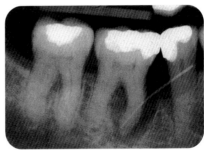

ment plan to include either root canal treatment or extraction of the affected tooth. Testing should be done using at least two methods – commonly application of ethyl chloride and an electric pulp tester – as false positives and negatives are common. This is true especially in elderly patients whose teeth have large amounts of secondary dentine and for a similar reason in heavily restored teeth. The contra-lateral and adjacent teeth should also be routinely tested as controls. If results of vitality testing are equivocal, preparation of a test cavity is ultimately the acid test. If the tooth is still vital the patient will respond as the amelo-dentinal junction of the tooth is broached by the bur and a small restoration should subsequently be placed. If the patient does not respond, the operator can be confident that the tooth is non-vital and progress to root canal therapy or extraction. A common reason for individual sites being unresponsive to periodontal therapy is due to pocket re-infection from organisms of endodontic origin.

3. Use of a gutta percha point to track back to the source of infection. When a patient presents with a sinus, it is not always straightforward to decide upon the source of the problem, as infection will track along the path of least resistance. Identification of the source is especially difficult if there

is generalised periodontal disease and the dentition is heavily restored. However, isolation of the cause is an essential prerequisite if appropriate therapy is to begin. One useful method is to introduce a gutta percha point into the sinus and gently explore it back along the sinus tract until resistance is felt. If a radiograph is taken at this time with the point in place, the source of the infection is often located at the site at which the point lies (Fig 9-20).

4. Use of study models. These are useful in cases with occlusal problems and particularly in those demonstrating tooth migration. They are valuable not just singly but as a series, where models are produced at repeated intervals. Models display changes over a period of time and if the changes are small but continuous they could be missed if clinical evaluation alone was used. Comparison of an early model with one from later in the series often shows such changes very clearly and is useful in alerting the clinician to the prospect that active treatment rather than just monitoring of a situation may be required. The models are also useful in treatment planning and later may be used to check the progress of treatment and to act as a baseline for maintenance regimes.

5. Use of photographs. A photographic record is often extremely useful either on its own or as an addition to study models. Again, a series of photographs is a great addition to the written description and this record provides valuable baseline information and shows progress over time, particularly for soft tissue lesions.

6. Gingival biopsy. This is useful in some cases to confirm a diagnosis although interpretation of the tissue histology produced is often made more difficult by the omnipresence of gingival inflammation. The biopsy site chosen and the technique used should also be carefully considered as any defect in the gingival contour is extremely unaesthetic and may promote plaque accumulation. When there is suspicion that the lesion may be malignant, an incisional biopsy is necessary, so that if the lesion is confirmed as such, the original position and landmarks are still present for wider excision. Excisional biopsies are indicated for clearly benign lesions.

7. Tests to predict periodontal disease. The problem with virtually all clinical periodontal tests is that they are retrospective in nature – that is they confirm that disease has taken place and help the investigator measure how much has occurred, but do not provide information on current disease activity. The ultimate hope is for the development of a test which is cheap, simple and quick to perform, that will reliably predict patients at risk of future disease. Many studies during the 1980s and 1990s focused on markers of current or future disease activity measured within GCF. Whilst many achieved 70%-80% predictivity for future disease activity, such tests

were cumbersome and impractical for chair-side use and have never taken off. Theoretically, predictive tests would allow targeting of scarce resources at risk subjects such that initial screening would, one hopes, identify disease at an early stage and prevent or at least minimise disease progression. This would keep treatment needs simple and would thus increase the chance of the therapy being successful.

Many areas of research have been and currently are being investigated. The emphasis recently has moved in the direction of genetic testing. Several genetic polymorphisms have been described in the Interleukin-1 gene cluster (see Chapters 3 and 4) and associations have been reported between some of these and increased severity of several chronic inflammatory diseases including periodontitis. A peripheral blood "finger prick" test designed to detect these polymorphisms is now available, but its utility appears limited to predicting periodontal disease in non-smokers aged between 40 and 60 years of age, and only within certain demographic areas. It does not appear effective for all UK populations.

It seems unlikely that genetic tests will be perfect predictors for periodontitis, owing to the multi-factorial nature of the periodontal diseases. The attraction of genetic testing is that it is a once-in-a-lifetime test and would genuinely facilitate the establishment of truly preventive management programmes. There are many potential pitfalls with genetic testing as a whole and before we try to associate genetic markers with different periodontal diseases we need to be in agreement about what constitutes a particular disease. Unless we can agree clear clinical criteria (classifications) for a disease, we cannot investigate which genes, or polymorphisms of those genes, are linked to that disease.

Referral of Patients

Referral to a specialist should always be considered if a case is complicated because the clinical problem is unusual or difficult and/or the patient has a relevant medical condition. Deciding which cases to refer appropriately can be difficult and the reader should consult "Referral Policy and Parameters of Care" published by the British Society of Periodontology in October 2000 (www.bsperio.org).

Important Changes in Radiology

In the mid-1990s, the National Radiology Protection Board (NRPB) issued a statement on the use of ionising radiation during pregnancy. It may be concluded from this that the normal selection criteria for dental radiography do not need to be influenced by the possibility of a female patient being at any stage of pregnancy. In addition, there is no justification for the routine use of lead aprons for patients undergoing dental radiography – in fact their use during panoramic radiography is positively discouraged. Further information on these and related matters is available from the NRPB documents "Guidelines on Radiology Standards for Primary Dental Care Report by the Royal College of Radiologists and the National Radiological Protection Board" published in 1990 and "Guidance Notes for Dental Practitioners on the Safe Use of X-ray Equipment" published in 2001 (www.nrpb.org). Additional discussion of these issues will be found in a forthcoming book in the *Quintessentials* series, *21st-Century Imaging*.

Further Reading

Eley BM, Cox SW. Advances in periodontal diagnosis 1. Traditional clinical methods of diagnosis. Br Dent J 184;1998:12-16.

Eley BM, Cox SW. Advances in periodontal diagnosis 2. New clinical methods of diagnosis. Br Dent J 184;1998:71-74.

Guidelines on Radiology Standards for Primary Dental Care Report by the Royal College of Radiologists and the National Radiological Protection Board. National Radiology Protection Board. 1990.

Guidance Notes for Dental Practitioners on the Safe Use of X-ray Equipment. National Radiology Protection Board. 2001.

Referral Policy and Parameters of Care. British Society of Periodontology, 2000 (www.bsperio.org).

Chapter 10

Periodontal Diagnosis and Prognosis

Aim

This chapter aims to draw together the preceding text to enable practitioners to arrive at a practical working diagnosis upon which to develop appropriate treatment plans. (For further discussion of this see *Quintessentials: Treatment Planning for the Periodontal Team*.)

Outcome

Having read this chapter the reader should be able confidently to diagnose the majority of the more common periodontal diseases and to add detail to that diagnosis specific to the individual patient. The reader should also be able, on an individual patient basis, to identify local and systemic risk factors and to form an opinion about the degree of risk of future disease progression.

Diagnosis

Reaching a diagnosis and entering it in signed and dated patients' records should be routine practice. This should occur after the examination is completed when the patient first attends for treatment and should then be repeated at all subsequent re-evaluation appointments during maintenance.

A diagnosis should be a concise description of the presenting disease in a particular mouth at a particular time. It is useful both on its own and in a comparative way over a period of time. Changes in severity and distribution of disease over time are often highlighted in this way giving an indication of rate of change as well as just the degree of change seen. Since the best indicator for future periodontal disease in a patient is their past disease experience, this information is very valuable.

Possible Periodontal Diagnoses

In the past, people tended to talk about periodontal disease as though it was just one disease entity. Over the years, however, there has been recognition that there are many different forms of periodontal disease, which just happen to affect the same tissues. These can be differentiated in a number of ways including the ages of the patients involved, the severity, type and distribution of destruction seen and the presence of systemic involvement. Classification of periodontal diseases is discussed in detail in Chapter 6, but when considering plaque-induced inflammatory periodontal diseases three main diagnostic situations arise:

1. A stable periodontium. This diagnosis is consistent with clinical health and is made if all the pockets are shallow enough to be cleaned by the patients themselves (usually taken to mean pocket depths of ≤ 3mm) *and* there is no bleeding from the base of the pockets upon gentle probing. This is the ideal situation since:

   • there is no evidence of the inflammation which we know often precedes and accompanies periodontal breakdown

   • the patient should be able to maintain low plaque scores – it is to be hoped below their own individual disease threshold.

   If a patient presents in this condition no treatment is required and it is reasonable to conclude that their susceptibility to periodontal disease is probably relatively low. Sometimes, however, patients with higher susceptibility who have undergone successful periodontal therapy may also present in this way during periodontal maintenance. It is known that periodontal treatment does not change the innate susceptibility to periodontal disease of any patient. However, with adequate therapy and good co-operation the disease may be controlled. In such cases presentation with a stable periodontium is a welcome finding, but there must be recognition that the disease is never cured and continued vigilance in the form of an appropriate individually designed maintenance programme is required.

2. Gingivitis. This term means that there is no loss of attachment present (hence any pockets present must be false pockets), but there is redness, swelling and bleeding on probing from the base of the pockets, following gentle probing. As discussed in Chapter 5, it is known that gingivitis is the first stage of periodontal disease and that some patients never progress beyond this. Unfortunately, other patients with higher susceptibility to periodontal disease progress rapidly through gingivitis and quickly develop periodontitis. There are two main descriptors which should be applied to gingivitis to provide a clearer diagnostic picture. These are:

   • Whether the condition is *acute* or *chronic*. There is a great deal of confusion about these terms. It has often been assumed that "acute" means that the condition being described is severe in nature while "chronic" implies lower severity. The terms correctly, however, describe the length of time for which the condition has been present, with acute meaning for a short time and chronic describing a greater duration (see Chapter 6). There is no doubt that the terminology can be confusing, but in periodontal terms acute forms of gingivitis may include conditions such as NUG, primary herpetic gingivostomatitis or lateral periodontal abscesses. However, as previously discussed, such conditions may, more rarely, also follow a chronic course and the majority of gingivitis cases fall into one of the chronic gingivitis categories.

- Whether the condition is *localised* or *generalised*. There are no hard and fast rules about the differentiation between the two but the 1999 World Workshop on Periodontal Disease Classification suggests that the term "localised" be used if up to 30% of the mouth is affected and "generalised" if more than this figure is involved. A description of the affected teeth and surfaces involved in the localised form of the condition may be included. This addition is not necessary when the condition is generalised.

An example of a diagnosis would thus be "localised chronic gingivitis (affecting all surfaces of the lower incisors and canines)".

3. Periodontitis. This term is applied when there is loss of attachment resulting in the presence of *true* pockets *and* bleeding from the base of the pockets following gentle probing. The loss of attachment suffered means that the periodontal damage is, by definition, irreversible, though this does not mean that the condition cannot be stabilised. In this case three descriptors can be applied to the term periodontitis to maximise the clarity of the diagnosis.

- *Which type of periodontitis is present*. The classification system for this is discussed in Chapter 6 and the descriptions found there should enable the clinician to decide which form of periodontitis is present. The vast majority of patients presenting for treatment have chronic periodontitis. Even the *aggressive* forms of periodontitis are chronic conditions, *not* acute.

- *Whether the condition is localised or generalised*. The 30% rule is a guide, but is somewhat arbitrary, so common sense in the application of this term is recommended.

- *The severity of the condition*. There are no hard and fast rules here either and there are many suggestions about defining whether disease is mild, moderate or severe. Using a system is useful, however, as the descriptive words "mild", "moderate" and "severe", though intentionally useful, may mean entirely different things to different clinicians. Two measurements used to aid description of the severity are the clinical measure of LOA and radiographic evidence of *bone loss,* and the following is a suggestion of how severity may be described.

- *mild disease*: LOA of 1-2mm or loss of the bone covering up to one-third of the root length.
- *moderate disease*: LOA of 3-4mm or bone loss of up to one-half the root length
- *severe disease*: LOA of 5+mm or bone loss greater than one-half of the root and/or inclusion of furcation involvement.

Some systems use pocket depth as a means of defining disease severity, but as discussed earlier there is an in-built problem in using this measurement on its own, since it will not differentiate between true and false pockets and may thus markedly over- or underestimate the disease present.

An example of a diagnosis would be "generalised moderate chronic periodontitis", though it can be further refined by the addition of more detail, e.g. "generalised moderate chronic periodontitis with localised severe disease affecting the lower incisors and canines". This diagnosis actually means something and can be changed at a later date to reflect changes in the behaviour of the disease, its distribution or severity.

Prognosis

After diagnosis of periodontal disease many patients, perfectly reasonably, ask about their periodontal prognosis. In response, the clinician must necessarily be fairly guarded because the prognosis is basically the clinician's "best guess" about what is likely to happen based upon his/her knowledge and experience. The uncertainty of the situation arises at this stage because two vital factors are unknown:

- *The biological tissue response to treatment*. This can vary greatly from one patient to another and is sometimes surprising in that severe conditions may respond well, while apparently more trivial conditions show a poor response.
- *Patient co-operation*. The higher the innate susceptibility to periodontal disease the more important becomes the patient's co-operation. If this is poor, treatment will not succeed and this fact must be recognised by both the patient and the clinician. No matter how good the professional care may be, it cannot compensate for poor home care.

It is possible to give a prognosis, however, by consideration of certain general and local prognostic factors.

General Prognostic Factors

1. *The systemic health and immune status of the patient.* This is important, as it is known that many systemic conditions have negative consequences for the periodontium. Examples include many haematological, gastro-intestinal and endocrine diseases. Presence of such conditions may reduce the prognosis. Drugs taken by many patients to control their systemic disease may also adversely affect the periodontium. Examples include cytotoxic and immunosuppressive medication and certain drugs such as phenytoin, which may have the undesired side effect of causing gingival overgrowth (see Chapter 4).

2. *Heredity.* The role of genetics in many forms of periodontal disease is difficult to evaluate because periodontal diseases are polygenic, with many confounding environmental factors (e.g. smoking) influencing underlying genetic susceptibility. There is evidence of a significant role for genetic transmission in several types of periodontitis, in particular in some of the aggressive forms. It is always worth asking patients whether there is a family history of periodontal disease and this is especially worthwhile if the patient has presented with aggressive/severe disease.

3. *The aetiology and form of periodontitis.* Clearly the more aggressive the type of periodontal disease present the lower the prognosis.

4. *The age of the patient in relation to the attachment loss.* This encompasses the concept of susceptibility. If the patient is young and has good plaque control yet has severe disease it is clear that the prognosis is much poorer than if a similar level of destruction was seen in an elderly patient with poor plaque control. The clinician should specifically consider the innate susceptibility of *each* patient to periodontal disease, as this cannot be changed by treatment. In general, the higher the susceptibility the lower the prognosis will be, the more aggressive the treatment is likely to have to be and the shorter recall times must be if and when the disease is controlled.

5. *Whether the patient is a smoker.* There is now mounting and convincing evidence for the highly destructive effect of smoking on the periodontium (see Chapters 4 and 7). Smoking certainly reduces the periodontal prognosis.

6. *The attitude and co-operation of the patient.* There is no doubt that a successful outcome from periodontal treatment is dependent upon patient co-operation and that this becomes more important in patients with a high innate susceptibility to periodontal disease. Poor compliance will reduce prognosis in susceptible cases.

7. *The availability of treatment modalities.* There are many new forms of, or adjuncts to, periodontal therapy and the application of some in particular

circumstances may positively affect the prognosis. (For further discussion please see *Quintessentials: Treatment Planning for the Periodontal Team* and *Non-Surgical Management of Inflammatory Periodontal Diseases*.)

8. *The knowledge and experience of the clinician*. This does not mean that specialists should provide all periodontal care, but if the disease found is severe or complicated in any way, consideration should be given to referral of the patient to someone with specialist knowledge and skills.

9. *Institution of an adequate maintenance programme*. Periodontal disease cannot be cured and can at best be stabilised. As the innate susceptibility of a patient to their disease remains unchanged after treatment, even if the disease is controlled, it is possible – and in some cases likely – that the disease will recur. A good maintenance programme is required so that any such recurrence can be detected early while the treatment needs remain simple. Failure to institute a flexible, competent and individually designed maintenance plan will certainly reduce the long-term prognosis.

Local Prognostic Factors

1. *The amount of plaque present*. The plaque control in an individual mouth is adequate if the plaque level lies below the individual disease threshold for that patient and disease is controlled. Adequate control is thus a very individual concept and relates directly to the susceptibility of the individual to his or her own plaque. If the plaque control is inadequate the prognosis is reduced. This concept supports the *Non-Specific Plaque Hypothesis*.

2. *The organisms present in plaque*. There is compelling evidence that certain plaque bacteria such as *Actinobacillus actinomycetemcomitans* are particularly virulent (see Chapter 2). These organisms are described as having "a low critical infection", meaning that relatively few are required to cause a problem. Their presence reduces the prognosis and this concept supports the *Specific Plaque Hypothesis*.

3. *Pocket depth and location*. The deeper the pocket the more difficult it is to treat and the poorer the prognosis. The location of the pocket is also relevant as the ease of access reduces further back in the mouth. The access is thus least restricted in the anterior segments and the prognosis is generally improved in these sites.

4. *Amount and expanse/distribution of loss of attachment*. These are clearly negatively related to prognosis.

5. *Presence and severity of furcation involvement*. This is negatively related to prognosis (see Chapter 8).

6. *The restorative condition*. The presence of poor restoration margins, poorly designed dentures and orthodontic appliances will all tend to reduce the

prognosis as they make achieving adequate plaque control difficult if not virtually impossible.

7. *The endodontic condition.* If a tooth has both endodontic and periodontal involvement its prognosis is reduced, as it will need to be either extracted or have successful root canal therapy (RCT) performed before the periodontal work can begin. The chance of successful RCT is reduced in its own right by many factors including location within the mouth, root curvature, presence of obstructions in the canal, etc. (For further discussion see *Quintessentials: Managing Pulp Canal Infection*).

8. *The activity of the periodontal disease.* The more active sites present the lower the prognosis.

9. *The root length.* If the roots are short, a given number of millimetres of bone loss or loss of attachment is relatively much more serious than if the roots are long. Short-rooted teeth thus tend to have a lower prognosis than similar teeth with longer roots.

10. *The root shape.* The presence of root grooves and furrows promotes plaque accumulation and reduces prognosis in susceptible patients.

11. *Anomalies of tooth position.* Crowding or tilting of teeth can increase plaque accumulation and reduce the effectiveness of plaque control measures resulting in reduced prognosis in susceptible patients.

12. *Presence of calculus.* Although calculus is inert, it has a rough surface, which promotes plaque accumulation, which in a susceptible patient will reduce prognosis.

Consideration of all the above will allow the clinician to give a reasoned response to the issues of accurate periodontal diagnosis and prognosis.

Further Reading

Lindhe J, Karring T, Lang NP (Eds.) Clinical Periodontology and Implant Dentistry. 3rd ed. Copenhagen: Munksgaard, 1998.

Manson JD, Eley BM (Eds.) Outline of Periodontics. 4th ed. Oxford: Wright, 2000.

Index

Quintessentials for General Dental Practitioners Series

in 36 volumes

Editor-in-Chief: Professor Nairn H F Wilson

The Quintessentials for General Dental Practitioners Series covers basic principles and key issues in all aspects of modern dental medicine. Each book can be read as a stand-alone volume or in conjunction with other books in the series.

	Publication date, approximately
Oral Surgery and Oral Medicine, Editor: John G Meechan	
Practical Dental Local Anaesthesia	available
Practical Oral Medicine	Spring 2004
Practical Conscious Sedation	Autumn 2003
Practical Surgical Dentistry	Spring 2004
Imaging, Editor: Keith Horner	
Interpreting Dental Radiographs	available
Panoramic Radiology	Autumn 2003
Twenty-first Century Dental Imaging	Autumn 2004
Periodontology, Editor: Iain L C Chapple	
Understanding Periodontal Diseases: Assessment and Diagnostic Procedures in Practice	available
Decision-Making for the Periodontal Team	Autumn 2003
Successful Periodontal Therapy – A Non-Surgical Approach	Autumn 2003
Periodontal Management of Children and Adolescents	Autumn 2003
Periodontal Medicine in Practice	Spring 2004
Implantology, Editor: Lloyd J Searson	
Implants for the General Practitioner	available
Managing Orofacial Pain in General Dental Practice	Spring 2003

Endodontics, Editor: John M Whitworth

Rational Root Canal Treatment in Practice	available
Managing Endodontic Failure in Practice	Autumn 2003
Managing Dental Trauma in Practice	Autumn 2003
Managing the Vital Pulp in Practice	Autumn 2004

Prosthodontics, Editor: P Finbarr Allen

Teeth for Life for Older Adults	available
Complete Dentures – from Planning to Problem Solving	Autumn 2003
Removable Partial Dentures – A Systematic Approach	Autumn 2003
Fixed Prosthodontics for the General Dental Practitioner	Autumn 2003
Occlusion: A Theoretical and Team Approach	Autumn 2004

Operative Dentistry, Editor: Paul A Brunton

Decision-Making in Operative Dentistry	available
Applied Dental Materials in Operative Dentistry	Spring 2003
Aesthetic Dentistry	Autumn 2003
Successful Indirect Restorations in General Practice	Spring 2004

Paediatric Dentistry/Orthodontics, Editor: Marie Therese Hosey

Child Taming: How to Cope with Children in Dental Practice	Spring 2003
Paediatric Cariology	Autumn 2003
Treatment Planning for the Developing Dentition	Autumn 2003

General Dentistry and Practice Management, Editor: Raj Rattan

The Business of Dentistry	available
Risk Management in General Dental Practice	Spring 2003
Practice Management for the Dental Team	Autumn 2003
Application of Information Technology in General Dental Practice	Spring 2004
Quality Assurance in General Dental Practice	Autumn 2004
Evidence-Based Care in General Dental Practice	Spring 2005

Quintessence Publishing Co. Ltd., London

Page 64

69   dibeties

112   تَصِيُر probes

122   تَصِوير

151